Food Policy

Series editors

Martin Caraher, London, UK
John Coveney, Adelaide, Australia

More information about this series at http://www.springer.com/series/13344

John Coveney • Sue Booth

Editors

Critical Dietetics and Critical Nutrition Studies

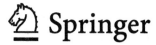 Springer

Editors
John Coveney
Flinders University
Adelaide, SA, Australia

Sue Booth
Flinders University
Adelaide, SA, Australia

ISSN 2365-4295   ISSN 2365-4309   (electronic)
Food Policy
ISBN 978-3-030-03112-1   ISBN 978-3-030-03113-8   (eBook)
https://doi.org/10.1007/978-3-030-03113-8

Library of Congress Control Number: 2019930085

This Springer imprint is published by the registered company Springer Nature Switzerland AG
The registered company address is: Gewerbestrasse 11, 6330 Cham, Switzerland

Introduction

It takes real bravery for a profession to turn inwards and critically examine aspects of professional training and practice. Speaking on bravery, Buddhist nun Pema Chodron notes we should "lean into the sharp points and fully experience them. The essence of bravery is being without deception".[1] So, what then are the sharp points for contemporary dietetics? Our contributing authors explore the rough edges and offer a range of unflinching perspectives on how critical dietetics can be used to ask important and, at times, uncomfortable questions. It is only by questioning and reflecting that we can advance and ensure the practice of dietetics remains relevant. This unique book brings together an edited collection of chapters exploring the critical dietetics landscape, what it looks like, feels like and smells like in real life. Without doubt, the chapters in this book foreshadow authentic, and socially just rewards may come from exploring new ways of being in the profession.

The book's *opening chapter* examines the genesis of the critical dietetics movement by Jacqui Gingras and Jennifer Brady. The chapter traces the events and circumstances of the movement's origins in Canada. Practitioner insights and early impacts from the fledgling movement are provided along with a future vision. In Chap. 2, Brady and Gingras introduce the value, theories and methods of critical dietetics and their value with respect to practice, advocacy and activism. The three tenets of critical dietetics axiology (anti-oppression, critical praxis and reflexivity) are introduced to provide clarity of the movement's underpinning values.

The next two chapters (3 and 4) turn to examine dietetic training and education with the goal of producing graduate dietitians that can thrive in the twenty-first century. In moving from the profession's roots in home economics and into health-care professionals, we have grasped the biomedical approach with both hands at the expense of more humanistic approaches to practice. Writing in Chap. 3, MacLellan suggests that in the current educational paradigm, "new dietitians are not ready for the relational and messy aspects of our work". Changes to underlying belief systems are needed in order to produce new innovative practices that challenge the status quo.

---

[1] Chodron P. (2001) *The Places that Scare You: A Guide to Fearlessness in Difficult Times.* Shambhala Press.

In Chap. 4, Lordly reflects on the shortcomings of traditional top-down, positivist academic dietetic training. In order to re-engineer a critical dietetic approach to practice, educators need to provide safe spaces, relinquish their power as experts and foster opportunities for knowledge co-creation and reflexivity.

Occupational and positional power of dietetic practitioners within a clinical setting is explored in Chap. 5. Here, Morley provides insight into the nature of various power dynamics and suggests that in order to bring a client-centred focus to our work, we need to embrace connectivity, rich dialogue and knowledge co-production to transform and inform critical dietetic practice. Implicit in this chapter and the specific clinical setting is an appreciation of multidisciplinary approaches (of other health-care/medical specialists) and commitments to both reflexive practice and the co-production of knowledge with clients and colleagues.

The book moves to the food system, its imperialism and impact on population health and our environment. There are synergies between Chap. 6 by Booth and Coveney and Chap. 7 by Carlsson et al. which comes later. Booth and Coveney briefly introduce the concept of food democracy as a way that consumers can take back some control of the food system through their own food choices and experiences. With its roots in civic agriculture, civic dietetics is a way of reorienting professional practice. By embracing roles as navigators, whistle-blowers and advocates, dietetic practice may be more aligned with the tenets of critical dietetics.

Carlsson, Mehta and Petinger begin Chap. 7 by highlighting historical engagement of the nutrition and dietetic community with food system sustainability. The chapter then moves to define foundational concepts of sustainability in food systems and diets, from a systems perspective. The chapter shows how some of today's pressing nutritional challenges are sustainability challenges and examples of the interface between today's dietetics and food system sustainability. The chapter ends with a discussion on the role of nutrition and dietetic practitioners in food system sustainability and the needs and challenges for dietetic education to support that role.

Using different ways of knowing food and the different appreciation of what is "good" food, Coveney in Chap. 8 explores some of the ethical considerations associated with dietetic practices. The scientific principles that underpin the theories of dietetics are often at odds with tradition and culture, which privilege other forms of knowing. In their roles as providers of expert advice on food and health, dietitians often have to walk a tight line between science and gastronomy: that is science and art of food and eating. The chapter shows how using the critical dietetics lens allows for a more nuanced understanding of ways of appreciating food.

In Chap. 9, White traces the development of the history of American food system, where food production is driven purely by profit. Such capitalistic approaches have serious consequences for human health, food and water safety, the environment, loss of agricultural communities and various forms of oppression. Alternative approaches such as urban agriculture and sustainable farming offer hope for a more equitable and accessible food system.

The potential role of dietitians as advocates mentioned in earlier chapters (especially 6 and 7) is explored in more detail by Brady in Chap. 10. The question posed is "How dietetic practitioners can extend their roles be social health equity advocates for those affected by disadvantage?" A highlight of this chapter is the two case studies of dietitians using their position and privilege and striving for a fairer, more just world. This strongly aligns with the idea implicit in the critical dietetics framework that practice positions should be just and socially accountable.

Contents

About the Authors

Sue Booth is an academic at Flinders University in the College of Medicine and Public Health. Sue teaches into the Masters of Public Health Programme and has published in the areas of food insecurity and food systems.

Jennifer Brady is an assistant professor in Applied Human Nutrition at Mount Saint Vincent University. Her work draws on critical and feminist theory to explore food, nutrition, health and expertise.

Liesel Carlsson lectures in the School of Nutrition and Dietetics at Acadia University and is a PhD candidate in Strategic Sustainable Development at the Blekinge Institute of Technology in Sweden. In her teaching, she works to integrate a sustainability lens into all aspects of food and nutrition learning. She publishes on and is actively involved in school gardens, sustainable food in institutions and engaging communities in global sustainability goals. She co-chairs the Dietitians of Canada Sustainable Food Systems Leadership Team.

John Coveney is a professor of global food, culture and health at Flinders University. He is an accredited practising dietitian (Australia) and holds state registration in dietetics in the UK. John has published over 200 articles and sole authored several books and book chapters on food, culture and health.

Jacqui Gingras is an associate professor in the Department of Sociology at Ryerson University. Her research and teaching involves theoretical and experiential explorations of health epistemology, health activism and social movements. She has published in the *Fat Studies Journal*, *Journal of Sociology* and *Critical Public Health*. She is the founding editor of the *Journal of Critical Dietetics*, an open-access, peer-reviewed journal at http://criticaldietetics.ryerson.ca.

Daphne Lordly is a registered dietitian (Nova Scotia) and a member of Dietitians of Canada (DC). She holds a NSDA Honorary Lifetime Membership and has received a DC Fellow Award. Her research interests include dietetic education, in particular the socialization of dietetic students and practitioners with an emerging interest in how gender is implicated in these processes and arts-informed research and pedagogy.

Elin Lövestam is an associate senior lecturer in the Department of Food Studies, Nutrition and Dietetics, Uppsala University. She is a registered dietitian in Sweden, and her main research and teaching interests consider the professional approach and role of the dietetic practitioner.

Debbie MacLellan is currently the president of the University of Canada in New Cairo, Egypt. She spent 28 years at the University of Prince Edward Island in Charlottetown, Prince Edward Island as a professor, dean of science and co-chair of the Strategic Planning Committee in the president's office. She was a registered dietitian for almost 40 years and a dietetic educator for 28 years.

Kaye Mehta is Head of Teaching Section and Domain Leader for Public Health and Community Nutrition in Nutrition and Dietetics. She brings more than 30 years of practice experience in community nutrition in Adelaide and cultivates strong partnerships with community organizations in her teaching and research. Her expertise spans nutritional ecology, programme evaluation and a justice approach to working with community.

Catherine Morley is an associate professor in the School of Nutrition and Dietetics at Acadia University. She is registered with the Nova Scotia Dietetic Association and a life member and fellow of dietitians of Canada. Catherine's research interests are how developing an understanding of the lived experiences of eating with changed health status or life circumstances informs approaches to nutrition education and counselling; arts in dietetic practice, education and research; and dietetics history.

Clare Pettinger is a Registered Dietitian and Registered Nutritionist (Public Health) and lecturer at the University of Plymouth, UK. She is actively engaged in research on "sustainability for dietitians" and "food justice." As an inspired educator, she frequently acts as an advocate for sustainable eating and believes strongly that new approaches are required to tackle current local (and global) health and social wellbeing challenges.

Jillian Ruhl is currently completing her dietetic internship to become a registered dietitian in Canada. Her research interests include the dietetic student experience, and the intersection between dietetics, art, agriculture and foods studies.

Jill H. White Jill White is Associate Professor Emeritus at Dominican University, where she continues to teach online and administrate a Head Start Nutrition Grant with the City of Chicago. Her clinical experiences as a Pediatric Dietitian centered around the South Side of Chicago where she began her academic career precepting students from Chicago internships, including Malcolm X College Dietetic Technology Program.

Chapter 1
The History of Critical Dietetics: The Story of Finding Each Other

Jacqui Gingras and Jennifer Brady

> *The most important thing is that we found each other, Jill White.*
> *(member, Critical Dietetics, 2018)*

Aim of Chapter and Learning Outcomes

The primary aim of this chapter is to provide context for the historical development of Critical Dietetics.

At the end of this chapter, readers will be able to

- Discuss the historical context for why and how critical dietetics emerged
- Recall the events that lead to the development of critical dietetics over the last decade
- Describe the recollections of and impact on those who were present when critical dietetics originated and areas of exploration continue to exist for the movement

Summary

Critical Dietetics has emerged in the last decade as a response to a primarily positivist orientation to what is seen as acceptable knowledge in the field of dietetics. As more and more valid contributions were made from outside of this dominant orientation to professionals' and scientists' ways of knowing in food and nutrition, epistemologies shifted and enlarged. This process continues to unfold with the emergence of Critical Dietetics and now critical food and nutrition studies. While

J. Gingras (✉)
Department of Sociology, Ryerson University, Toronto, ON, Canada
e-mail: jgingras@ryerson.ca

J. Brady
Mount Saint Vincent University, Halifax, NS, Canada

© Springer Nature Switzerland AG 2019
J. Coveney, S. Booth (eds.), *Critical Dietetics and Critical Nutrition Studies*,
Food Policy, https://doi.org/10.1007/978-3-030-03113-8_1

1

these fields have not entirely merged in their efforts, those most closely involved with Critical Dietetics offer a vision for the future.

Introduction

Over the past 10 years, Critical Dietetics (CD) has emerged as a leading voice for critical research, practice, and education within dietetics and continues to grow. During this time CD has been strengthened with new members, an open-access journal, and a governance structure that will continue to build capacity within Critical Dietetics and to effect change within the dietetic profession. This chapter recounts the history of the movement and unfolds in five parts. First, we offer a brief account of the beginnings of CD. Second, we include a reprint of one of the founding documents of the movement, *Critical Dietetics: A Declaration*, which was first published as a post on Dietitians of Canada's blog, *Practice*. Third, Dr. Jacqui Gingras, chapter co-author and the person responsible for bringing together those who founded CD, offers a personal account and reflection on the creation and evolution of the movement. Fourth, we share reflections from other Critical Dietitians, namely, those who have been engaged with CD from the beginning and have ideas about what the movement has meant for them and what changes are needed for further growth. Finally, we offer some concluding remarks and thoughts for a vision for the future of CD.

The Origins of Critical Dietetics

In June 2009, a research workshop was held in the classrooms of Kerr Hall on the Ryerson University campus in Toronto, Ontario, Canada. The event was attended by a small number of scholars, practitioners, and students and represented the culmination of several months of effort by Dr. Jacqui Gingras, one of the authors of this chapter. Dr. Gingras secured a national grant from the Social Sciences and Humanities Research Council (SSHRC) to host a workshop that would bring together critical scholars, practitioners, and students. The title of the workshop was *Beyond Nutritionism: Rescuing Dietetics Through Critical Dialogue* (hereafter referred to as *Beyond Nutritionism*). It was at *Beyond Nutritionism*, through the collaboration of researcher, practitioner, and student participants, that Critical Dietetics was born. The intention to initiate a movement called Critical Dietetics was not the organizing feature of this gathering; however that is exactly what happened, and in looking back at the title of the workshop, both of the words "critical" and "dietetics" were there.

The purpose of *Beyond Nutritionism* was to bring together leading Canadian dietetic theorists, researchers, students, and practitioners along with international advisors to engage in critical dialogue that would enhance the social, cultural, and political relevance and resonance of dietetics. This workshop provided an opportunity for participants to identify and critique new fields of transdisciplinary research in the aforementioned areas, as well as to create and grow a viable international research network that would enhance capacity for culturally and socially relevant dietetic inquiry. More specifically, *Beyond Nutritionism* provided a space enabled for researchers, and practitioners, and students to explore the highly emergent and critical issues of gender, race, class, ability, and size in dietetics; dietetic epistemologies; post-structural orientations to dietetic education and practice; art-based inquiry within dietetics; empowerment, compliance, and the ethical subject in dietetics; and integration of dietetics with social justice, social responsibility, and the human right to food and health.

The workshop proposal outlined that 30 Canadian academic and practicing dietetic attendees would participate in the workshop, along with 3 international advisors from the USA, the UK, and Australia. Canadian participants were invited because of their leadership within the discipline and their desire to bring a critical dialogue to bear on the profession. International advisors were selected for their ability to hold a critical transdisciplinary lens to dietetics and hailed from sociology, disability studies, textile arts, gender studies, and education. The workshop facilitator, Leslie Bella, of Queen's University, was chosen because of her knowledge of the field as per her work on professionalization in healthcare professions, plus a wealth of experience in fostering critical dialogue and success at publishing. Also included among the attendees were students who were invited to submit a memorandum of interest related to the workshop topics. Five students were selected to present their full papers at the workshop. The workshop also included two observers who held stakeholder positions within the profession as representatives from Dietitians of Canada, the national association of dietitians in Canada, and the Ontario College of Dietitians, the regulatory body governing the practice of dietetics in the province of Ontario, Canada. Additional student project assistants assisted with the planning and implementation of the workshop. Event activities included paper presentation sessions, small group research circles, and working groups.

The sessions included paper presentations by three to four newer scholars and one experienced scholar who acted as a discussant to weave together the themes of the papers with their own thinking on the topic. Over 2 days, there were five sessions presented with titles such as "Learning to Not Know in Dietetics," "Releasing the Dietetic Imaginary," "Surfacing the Body in Dietetics," "Living an Audacious Curriculum," and "Making Possible a World Beyond Nutritionism." In total, there were 17 presenters and 5 discussants. Discussants included Marjorie DeVault, Ann Fox, Lucy Aphramor, John Coveney, and Jacqui Gingras. The paper presentations were interspersed with small group work to integrate and synthesize themes that arose, as well as to determine a communication plan and priorities for action. The vision for Critical Dietetics took shape during the facilitated whole group discussions. Some options for our future work together that emerged from the small and whole group discussions included collaborative research projects, conferences, and a journal. We also collectively determined near the end of the workshop that we were going to be called Critical Dietetics.

There were three main dissemination strategies for emerging Critical Dietetics work developed over the course of the 2-day *Beyond Nutritionism* workshop: (1) a peer-reviewed, edited book that would include papers presented at the workshop; (2) a new open-access journal for critical research in dietetics; and (3) a blog post for Dietitians of Canada's blog, *Practice*. These dissemination products, along with the workshop website, would integrate the workshop planning, communication, and papers to enable access by a wider audience of dietetic and other health professionals as well as interdisciplinary scholars and students. The target audiences for the scholarly and creative contributions to those dissemination products included researchers, practitioners, and students within the field of dietetics and related health profession such as nursing, social work, and early childhood education, as well as social science disciplines such as sociology, anthropology, and education. Soon after *Beyond Nutritionism*, the *Journal of Critical Dietetics* was established. Also, at the urging of Dr. Catherine Morley, who was the editor of the *Practice* blog at the time, we collaboratively wrote and published *Beyond Nutritionism: An Invitation to Critical Dietetics Dialogue* for the *Practice* blog which included *Critical Dietetics: A Declaration*. In the *Practice* blog post, we invited others to sign on to the Declaration and support the emerging Critical Dietetics movement. The *Practice* blog post was published on December 3, 2009, and is reprinted below. The *Practice* blog post also coincided with the preparation of another grant for support to host the first Critical Dietetics conference, which was held in June 2010, also in Toronto. A second SSHRC grant was received to support the hosting of the first conference.

Beyond Nutritionism built on existing lines of research while enhancing the capacity for dietetic research as it continued to grow in new, creative, and critical directions. A few years prior to *Beyond Nutritionism*, in 2005, the Canadian Association for Food Studies (CAFS) formed (Power and Koc 2008). A few years after *Beyond Nutritionism*, a group of scholars published a special issue of the academic journal, *Gastronomica* (Guthman 2014), in which they described the emerging field of critical nutrition studies. Since then, critical nutrition studies have continued to grow, and an edited volume, *Doing Nutrition Differently: Critical Approaches to Diet and Dietary Intervention*, was later published (Hayes-Conroy and Hayes-Conroy 2013). CAFS, and food studies more generally, share some interests with CD, namely, exploring critical perspectives of food and eating as social, cultural, political, and economic phenomena. Similarly, critical nutrition studies are concerned with the ways in which nutrition and nutrition intervention reflect discourses and relationships of power and are rooted in a theoretical tradition known as science and technology studies, or STS. Although CD shares some important common interests and political commitments with food studies and critical nutrition studies, CD is also unique in bringing together critical theoretical perspectives of health, food, and nutrition, with an aim to effect change through dietetic practice and advocacy.

Critical Dietetics: A Declaration
Thursday, December 3, 2009

Beyond Nutritionism: An Invitation to Critical Dietetics Dialogue
In spring of 2009, a research workshop entitled "Beyond Nutritionism: Rescuing Dietetics through Critical Dialogue" was held at Ryerson University and funded by the Social Sciences and Humanities Research Council. Appropriately, for a springtime gathering, it marked the establishment of a new movement – Critical Dietetics.

At the workshop, leading international theorists, researchers, practitioners, students, and advisors had long-awaited conversations regarding gender, race, class, ability, size, dietetic epistemology, post-structural orientations to dietetic education, art, and poetry in the context of dietetics. The result was an animated, groundbreaking commitment to redefine the profession through Critical Dietetics.

What counts as "knowing" in dietetic practice? How do we, as nutrition professionals, come to know what we don't know? How does the evidence-based culture of dietetics give voice? Where does dietetic culture render silence? What is it that we have already accomplished as a profession? In what ways do we continue to evolve? How can we further build upon the rich roots of our profession? What do we envision for the future of our profession? These are but a few of the difficult, essential questions that Critical Dietetics seeks to explore.

Critical Dietetics takes courage as we depart from familiar ways of doing and knowing. Indeed as Simmons (2009) challenged us in an earlier edition of Practice, it is time to "expand" (p. 3) our dietetic identities to become more "pluralistic" (p. 3), as we move beyond mere nutritionism (Pollan 2008) in our work.

Critical Dietetics requires conviction for change, comfort with the uncertainty of not knowing, acceptance of the blurry divide between art and science, and a desire for our allies' knowledge in social sciences, humanities, and natural sciences with whom we have much to integrate. We can grapple with the limits of science alongside the imperative to use it and venture into the vulnerability evoked by the merging of personal and professional ways of knowing. We are authors of our own experience and supportive witnesses to one another's growth in the midst of this new terrain.

Critical Dietetics: A Declaration stands as testament to the commitment the initial group has forged. It is extended as an invitation to our colleagues to become companion dietetic explorers in this exciting new movement. Together we can expand the body of knowledge in dietetics and shape the future of our profession.

Critical Dietetics: A Declaration – June 2009
Dietetics is a diverse profession with a commitment to, and tradition of, enhancing health, broadly defined, through diet and food. We recognize the commitment and hard work undertaken by dietetic professionals of the past and present who continue to innovatively shape and reshape the profession

from its roots in home economics to the incorporation of contemporary perspectives on health. While recognizing the multiple meanings of food and its power to nourish and heal, we acknowledge that food is more than the mere sum of its constituent nutrients. We recognize that human bodies in health and illness are complex and contextual. Moreover, we recognize that the knowledge that enables us to understand health is socially, culturally, historically, and environmentally constructed.

Building on the past century of dietetics and the "Beyond Nutritionism" workshop held at Ryerson University June 12–14, 2009, we extend an invitation to individuals in all areas of dietetic education, practice, and research to collaborate on the Critical Dietetics initiative.

Critical Dietetics is informed by transdisciplinary scholarship from the natural sciences, social sciences, and humanities. By contributing to scholarship, practice, and education, it strives to make visible our assumptions, give voice to the unspoken, embrace reflexivity, reveal and explore power relations, encourage public engagement and diverse forms of expression, and acknowledge that there are no value-free positions. Through these principles, Critical Dietetics will engage with the ever-changing health, social, and environmental issues facing humanity.

Assuming a critical stance means remaining inquisitive and willing to ask and hear challenging questions. Critical approaches grant us permission to imagine new ideas and explore new ways of approaching our practice. Critical Dietetics creates space for an emancipatory (i.e., liberating and socially just) scholarship by drawing upon many perspectives, philosophies, orientations, ways of asking questions, and ways of knowing.

Critical Dietetics derives its strength from supportive relationships, recognizing that it takes courage to step beyond familiar ways of knowing. It invites constructive dialogue and challenges us to discuss, debate, and rethink what we know and how we know it. It is a generative and collective effort which understands that strength comes from diversity and debate. This declaration is therefore a bold invitation that welcomes different ways of thinking and practicing within our own profession and in collaboration with allied fields. We anticipate collectively expanding the body of knowledge in dietetics and continuing the inclusive, scholarly, collective, and pluralistic development of the profession. If you want to contribute to this dialogue and become a signatory of Critical Dietetics, please email your expression of interest to jgingras@ryerson.ca by January 7, 2010.

Sincerely,

Lucy Aphramor (UK) BSc, RD
Yuka Asada MHSc, RD
Jennifer Atkins MHSc, RD

Mustafa Koc PhD
Esther Ignagni MSc
Daphne Lordly RD

Shawna Berenbaum PhD, RD, FDC
Jenna Brady BA, BASc, MHSc
Shauna Clarke (UK) BA, MA

John Coveney (Australia) MPHEd, PhD
Marjorie DeVault (USA) PhD
Lisa Forster-Coull MA, RD
Ann Fox MHSc, PhD, RD
Jacqui Gingras PhD, RD
Charna Gord MEd, RD

Debbie MacLellan PhD, RD, FDC
Elizabeth Manafo MHSc, RD
Catherine Morley MA, PhD, RD, FDC
Dean Simmons MSc(c), RD
Karen Trainoff BASc, RD
Roula Tzianetas MSc, RD
Jennifer Welsh MSc
Kristen Yarker-Edgar MSc, RD

Jacqui's Narrative

The date of the actual workshop was June 12–14, 2009, but the effort I put forward to secure the funding to host the event occurred much earlier during the year prior. I had been a tenure-track faculty member for only 2 years when the thought occurred to me "What would it be like to have the people in the same room who have inspired my questioning of this profession?" That is simply what I set out to do, bring as many of those people together as possible, invite them to share what remained to be said of dietetics, and see what came of it.

I decided to call the workshop *Beyond Nutritionism: Rescuing Dietetics Through Critical Dialogue* because I had recently been introduced to Scrinis' (2013) definition of nutritionism, and when thinking of the space I had hoped to create with the workshop, it was necessary to be explicit that the profession needed to go well beyond nutritionism, i.e., the singular focus on nutrients as a means to promote health. Nutritionism was our profession's safe and familiar space, and certainly there was more acknowledgment in our professional identity and practices. I was also influenced by Austin's (1999) work that stated dietitians and nutrition professionals were complicit in promoting low-fat foods to enhance the profit margins of the companies that produced such foods. I had always believed that we were more than just professional voices in collusion with corporations; I actually believed it was unethical for us to do so (Gingras 2005). I dreamed of a profession that was rooted in social justice, and I was unabashed in stating this publicly, and I also wanted to generate some disruptive tension in saying that the profession needed rescuing. I received comments about how the title was divisive and off-putting, but I did that intentionally to wake people up to a different way of doing dietetics. I believed that the people who needed to be at the workshop would be there regardless of what impact the name had more broadly.

The original list of attendees included Dr. Marjorie DeVault, a sociologist from Syracuse who was only one of two non-dietitians (Dr. Mustafa Koc being the second). Dr. DeVault (1999) wrote an influential study regarding how dietitians identify as activists, which resonated with me immediately. I invited those who had worked on other aspects of dietitian identity including Drs. Debbie MacLellan and Daphne Lordly, both of whom I had not met previously, although I had been well aware of their writing on the topic. After I had invited Dr. Catherine Morley who I had known for many years starting as my time as a dietetic intern, I had asked her who else should be on the guest list. Her first and most exuberant suggestion was Dr. John Coveney whose work, I admitted sheepishly, I had not encountered previously. "Well, it is about time you did!" she exclaimed. Now I am thankful that she shared his name and that he was able to participate. One attendee that I had connected with previously, but only by email, was Dr. Lucy Aphramor. During my doctoral studies, Dr. Aphramor reached out to me when my name was among the few that showed up on a Google search for feminist dietitians. *Beyond Nutritionism* would be the first time we would meet in person even after we had already initiated a prolific writing collaboration.

Students represented a significant group of participants from my point of view since I could see how the ideas shared at the workshop had potential to validate their experiences and ignite a powerful commitment to the movement. Of course, not all of the students that I had encountered thus far were open to questioning the profession; there were a few that indicated to me their desire to be part of what was happening. Those students were active members of the workshop as well as helping me as the local host and providing indispensable organizational supports. The other attendees commented that the student presence was significant and elevated the critical voice being expressed at *Beyond Nutritionism*.

Of note was the quality of the food that we ate. A local foodie, Laura Di Vilio, came with her own food truck, Di Vilio Good Food Co., and parked outside the workshop location and provided incredibly delicious, local, and nourishing meals and snacks for the entire group. I attribute the depth of our engagement in no small part to the food we enjoyed and the talk we experienced around the table.

There was intense resistance from my home department not to call the Declaration, "The Ryerson Declaration." I recall long conversations with Jennifer Welsh, a previous director of the department who was surprised by the resistance, but wanted to build on potential partnerships, and not isolate people, including many of her colleagues. At the time, I felt strongly that the name, Ryerson, should be closely associated with Critical Dietetics given that was where the movement originated; it offered an anchor or a placeholder to identify where the efforts began. The counter-argument was that because the workshop was organized by me and not one of my departmental colleagues was in support of it, the name of the university should not be used. I recall a brief, but frank email from a university executive indicating that it would be inappropriate to use the name Ryerson in this context and shortly after realized that it would indeed be better in the long run not to associate Critical Dietetics with one place, especially since I was one of the only academics associated with Ryerson that participated in the workshop, not including the majority of the students that attended. It was truly a blessing since it wasn't long after that I learned more about the colonial history of Egerton Ryerson who was the architect of indigenous residential schooling in Canada and, thus, almost 100 years of cultural genocide. Today the conversation continues about whether Ryerson University should change its name, so we were absolved of that burden when we were prevented from affiliating Critical Dietetics with Ryerson in the first place.

The Declaration served for an opening to those in the profession who were seeking that "missing piece" of criticality in their practice. It was a critical piece of writing to those attending *Beyond Nutritionism* that sought to acknowledge past contributions and not undermine those "discoveries." It was an important distinction for the authors of the Declaration to express; much good had come from the profession and from positivist nutrition science. The imperative underscoring that the Declaration made explicit was that positivist nutrition science, while significant, was not enough to explain the multiple ways of knowing what we had witnessed, experienced, and co-constituted during most of our careers as students, practitioners, and scholars to date. In other words, we felt that as a profession, we needed to appreciate the richness of meaning that food, nutrition, and health have for people, and to do that, we needed many lenses with which to view those things, only one of which was science. We believed it would be enough to express that acknowledgment publicly; by "… recogniz(ing) the commitment and hard work undertaken by dietetic professionals of the past and present," we would create a space for others to feel welcome. However, as has been written about previously (Gingras 2009), dietetics has unique challenges feeling seen within medical contexts and not generally open to critique. This dislocation (between positivist and interpretive "camps" within dietetics) remains difficult to bridge, but Critical Dietetics continues to invite dialogue on this thorny issue (Gingras et al. 2017).

Reflections from Critical Dietitians

This section allows for those who responded to questions we asked of them about their experiences at *Beyond Nutritionism*. The questions included asking workshop participants as well as those who may not have attended the workshop, but have been actively engaged since, about their expectations of the workshop, about their actual experience, and about their hopes and dreams for the future of Critical Dietetics. Questionnaire respondents gave permission for their real names to be used.

What Jacqui had hoped to provide for participants at *Beyond Nutritionism* was a supportive place for people and their ideas to flourish; it was an invitation to "go deeper into what dietetics is, has been, and could be" as Cathy Morley described. Several of those who participated in *Beyond Nutritionism* identified the environment to be surprisingly nonjudgmental and feeling-friendly; it was clear to Jacqui that such a space was necessary. She created an occasion for others that she had needed for herself. At the time of the workshop, Jacqui was experiencing resistance not only toward Critical Dietetics but toward her research program in general. This reality heightened the urgency for her to create a place for people to gather that offered collegial support. The fact that the workshop was held in the exact same classrooms in which Jacqui taught courses that invited open critique of the profession was symbolically empowering to her and others.

Although not experienced in the same way, many others had also expressed appreciation for being together with others that held similar views among which they had no need to "wear a mask" or to pretend to be someone who they thought the profession needed them to be in order to "fit." The idea that a mask would be necessary for a student or a dietetic practitioner is explored in other writings (Atkins and Gingras 2009; Brady et al. 2012; Gingras 2009, 2010; Good et al. 2016; Siswanto et al. 2014). Given the powerful cultural imperative that exists in dietetics to be other than one perceives her or himself to be, the notion of wearing a mask could be seen as a strategy for survival in our profession (Jordan 2017). Jordan (2017) explains that by "…keeping rejected aspects of (our)selves out of the relationship provides a sense of safety and lessens the overwhelming sense of vulnerability that accompanies rejection or a harsh response from another person" (p. 241). Sadly, this gesture is seen to be necessary by many in the dietetic profession.

In addition to being able to be authentic was the experience of having oft-marginalized research methods embraced, especially qualitative methods. Imagine the influence of having a life's work acknowledged as providing a meaningful contribution to the profession of which you were a member when previously it had not. As Lucy Aphramor described, "the discussions were often very emotionally intense, challenging, real…I felt vindicated for the times I had been treated as a nuisance/ridiculed etc because of speaking up." The profound sense of finally being seen and heard allowed attendees to do and say things that they had previously kept to themselves. For example, two attendees unrolled textile art they had created when they knew they were attending the workshop, and one student wrote and shared a poem he had written that was inspired during the sessions. Another talked about a dream she had the night before she was to present her paper that highlighted the violence she had felt she had been complicit in upholding through the internship process (Gingras and Brady with Aphramor 2014). Overall, what Debbie MacLellan wrote, "That workshop has had a powerful and lasting impact on the way I think about our profession and how I teach my students. I met people from a variety of backgrounds but who all had a common vision of doing nutrition differently. I loved that," was a sentiment that was shared by many in attendance.

Over the last eight years, Critical Dietetics has experienced many positive milestones such as the creation and publication of the *Journal of Critical Dietetics* and hosting of eight international Critical Dietetics conferences. The Journal has published seven issues and remains an open-access peer-reviewed journal. In much the same way that *Beyond Nutritionism* featured nontraditional methods of inquiry, so too does the *Journal of Critical Dietetics*. Work published includes art-based, storytelling, poetry, reflexive, and opinion. Plans are underway to promote the reach of this work and assess its impact on dietetic education and practice. The conferences continue to uphold the tradition established at *Beyond Nutritionism*, meeting with diverse groups of people in different parts of the world to share inspiring work that delves into often overlooked areas of education and practice within dietetics and nutrition. Just last summer we hosted our first strictly online conference that enabled many to attend at little cost to hear important work happening in different corners of practice. The commitment to have an online presence at each conference following was made to enable greater access and hopefully increased participation.

In addition to these successes, there are still many things left to explore such as establishing more robust partnerships with existing dietetic organizations such as the Academy of Nutrition and Dietetics in the USA and Dietitians of Canada, among others. Such a collaboration would assist both organizations in connecting with diverse audiences and providing more fulfilling supports to existing members. Becoming ever more politicized and reaching out and learning from people in different parts of the world who are practicing dietetics and have different perspectives to share is another long-term goal of Critical Dietetics if it wants to grow in socially relevant ways.

Conclusion and Imagineering

Berenbaum (2005) states that "We need imaginative and inventive dietitians to nourish dietetic practice, to move it forward. We need to think outside of the box, to take risks, to challenge the *status quo*" (p. 196). The creation of Critical Dietetics would not have been possible without imagination and our desire to take risks as a means to challenge the *status quo*. Those present at Beyond Nutritionism created Critical Dietetics as a means to enhance the dietetic profession even though, at times, some perceived we were trying to tear it down. In speaking about the difference between being critical (i.e., negative) and thinking critically, Berenbaum (2012) suggests that:

> All progressive professions should strive for, in fact EMBRACE, thinking critically, differently and deeply about their profession. Yes, at times we will be uncomfortable, confused, stressed or challenged. And that's ok. That's how it should be for a profession on the move. And at other times we will be inspired, excited, motivated, awed, reflective, and imaginative. (p. 2)

In thinking critically, we rely on many theories and constructs that we will expand upon in the next chapter in which we explore the foundations of Critical Dietetics axiology (core values of our movement). The work of creating a movement called Critical Dietetics isn't possible without borrowing from other thought leaders (theorists) who are also imaginative and deeply committed to shifting our view of the world forward. Finally, as we hope is abundantly clear by reading this chapter, Critical Dietetics emerged as a collective and collaborative endeavor. There are many people who were not present at the initial meetings that have contributed to the growth of this movement. And, now, through a process of organizational reform, Critical Dietetics is once again "on the move" with the hopes of drawing in a more diverse, international membership, including those from outside academia and those from the Global South. Such reform is sure to strengthen and further embolden Critical Dietetics in bringing a necessary and vital voice to the profession.

Assignments

1. Students in groups of 3–5 will watch a film from this list of documentaries (http://www.filmsforaction.org/articles/the-top-100-films-for-action/) and craft a manifesto for the social movement that is represented in the documentary. Each group will present to the class by sharing the title and the theme of the documentary and what they believe the documentary is trying to accomplish vis-à-vis their manifesto.
2. Invite students to write a 750-word narrative about a time in their lives when they changed their worldview. Each narrative is posted to a student blog, and each student is required to read at least two other entries and offer comment to the author about her/his experience.

Definition of Keywords and Terms

Critical	To be critical is to question the way things are so as to enhance or expand upon established epistemologies (ways of knowing) and bodies of knowledge. Often being critical is taken to be negative, but this is not a complete understanding. To be critical is to seek to transform and grow ways of thinking about any particular topic
Epistemology	Epistemology is a concept that describes the various ways of understanding what counts as knowledge. There are many epistemologies. Mainstream dietetic knowledge and practice are informed by positivist epistemology which understands knowledge creation as the process of uncovering truths about the world through the scientific method. Critical Dietetics is informed by a post-structural epistemology wherein truth is understood as being in constant flux and knowledge creation as requiring multiple, differently situated perspectives, approaches, and methods.
Nutritionism	Scrinis (2013) coined the term to describe the shifting focus toward the specific nutrients in food as providing some health benefits and the resulting emphasis by consumers to purchase food on this basis instead of other aspects such as taste, cost, or sociocultural meaning.
Transdisciplinary	This is the bringing together of different disciplines to offer a more complex and nuanced understanding of a topic, whereby the disciplines themselves are enhanced in the process. Transdisciplinary is different than multi- or interdisciplinary scholarship, in that the latter describes a process of bringing various disciplinary perspectives to bear on a topic, in this case, dietetic education, research, and practice, whereby dietetics is transformed and enhanced.

How This Chapter Addresses the Critical Dietetics Framework

This chapter adds a historical perspective that includes the multidisciplinary narratives of those who were responsible for founding the movement. The beginnings and development of CD lend vital context to the story of CD and to the other chapters included in the book. This chapter is rooted in the reflexive perspectives of those who participated in the meetings that initiated CD, as well as Jacqui Gingras' story, who was responsible for bringing together the group of people who founded CD. These individuals are sharing their narratives about the origins of CD, as well as their hopes for the future of the movement. This perspective includes a "looking back/looking forward" approach to the book, which is vital to provide the context necessary for reflexive thinking throughout the rest of the chapters and about the movement generally. As noted, the lived experiences of dietitians and the founders of CD are central to the chapter. This chapter includes the personal narrative of Jacqui Gingras, a former RD who paved the way for CD, as well as others who have been central to the development of CD. Socially-just policy and practice are the central commitments in our chapter. We tell the stories of those who led the way in bringing these new perspectives to dietetics. CD is responsible for creating platforms for the sharing of ideas related to social justice and dietetics. Telling these stories is important to documenting the history as context for the movement overall.

References

Atkins J, Gingras JR (2009) Coming and going: dietetic students' experiences of their education. Can J Diet Pract Res 70(4):181–186

Austin SB (1999) Commodity knowledge in consumer culture: the role of nutritional health promotion in the making of the diet industry. In: Sobal J, Maurer D (eds) Weighty issues: fatness and thinness as social problem. Aldine de Gruyter, New York, pp 159–181

Berenbaum B (2012) Who is a critical thinker? J Crit Diet 1(2):2

Berenbaum S (2005) Imagination nourishes dietetic practice: 2005 Ryley-Jeffs Memorial Lecture. Can J Diet Pract Res 66(3):193–196

Brady JL, Hoang A, Tzianetas R, Buccino J, Glynn K, Gingras J (2012) Unsuccessful dietetic internship applicants: a descriptive survey. Can J Diet Pract Res 73(2):e248–e252

DeVault M (1999) Whose science of food and health? Narratives of profession and activism from public health nutrition. In: Clarke AE, Olsen VL (eds) Revisioning women, health, and healing: feminist, cultural, and technoscience perspectives. Routledge, New York, pp 166–183

Gingras J (2005) Evoking trust in the nutrition counselor: why should we be trusted? J Agric Environ Ethics 18:57–74

Gingras J (2009) Longing for recognition: the joys, contradictions, and complexities of practicing dietetics. Raw Nerve Books, York

Gingras J (2010) The passion and melancholia of performing dietitian. J Sociol 46(4):437–453

Gingras J, Asada Y, Brady J, Aphramor L (2017) Critical dietetics: challenging the profession from within. In: Koc M, Sumner J, Winson A (eds) Critical perspectives in food studies, 2nd edn. Oxford University Press, Don Mills

Gingras J, Brady J with Aphramor L (2014) Harm has been done: ethical transgressions in becoming and being a dietitian. J Crit Diet 2(1):52–62

Good A, Brady J, Poultney M, Gingras J (2016) "Gatekeepers to the profession": exploring the experiences of Ontario dietetic internship coordinators. J Crit Diet 3(1):35–41

Guthman J (2014) Introducing critical nutrition: a special issue on dietary advice and its discontents. Gastronomica 14(3):1–4

Hayes-Conroy A, Hayes-Conroy J (eds) (2013) Doing nutrition differently: critical approaches to diet and dietary intervention. Ashgate, Surrey

Jordan J (2017) Relational–cultural theory: the power of connection to transform our lives. J Humanist Couns 56(3):228–224

Pollan M (2008) In defense of food: an eater's manifesto. The Penguin Press, New York

Power E, Koc M (2008) A double-double and a maple glazed doughnut. Food Cult Soc 11(3):263–267

Scrinis G (2013) Nutritionism: the science and politics of dietary advice. Columbia University Press, New York

Simmons D (2009) Questioning my dietitian identity. Practice 46:3

Siswanto O, Brady J, Alvarenga P, Magder A, Riesel J, Qureshi N, Gingras J (2014) Forgetting the pain: applicants' experiences of first-time success attaining a dietetic internship position in Ontario. J Crit Diet 2(1):45–51

Further Reading

Biltekoff C (2013) Eating right in America: the cultural politics of food and health. Duke University Press, Durham, NC

Travers KD (1997) Nutrition education for social change: critical perspective. J Nutr Educ 29:57–62

Chapter 2
Critical Dietetics: Axiological Foundations

Jennifer Brady and Jacqui Gingras

Aim of Chapter and Learning Outcomes

The aim of this chapter is to firstly introduce the core values, theories, and methods of Critical Dietetics and, secondly, to discuss the implications of the core values and theories for critical dietetic praxis within traditional practice areas as well as through advocacy and activism.

At the end of this chapter, readers will:

(i) Describe the core values, priorities, and tenets that guide critical dietetics
(ii) Define and discuss key terms and concepts that are important to the foundational values, theories, methods, and commitments of Critical Dietetics

Summary

In this chapter, we explore the core values of Critical Dietetics (CD) through three tenets, including a commitment to (1) anti-oppression, (2) critical praxis, and (3) reflexivity. We present these tenets as forming the basis of CD axiology, that is, the values of the CD movement. Through our discussion, we elaborate on several important facets of each tenet that give life and purpose to CD. These facets include the theoretical, epistemological, methodological, and pedagogical foundations and priorities that inform our work within the social health movement we are calling CD.

J. Brady (✉)
Applied Human Nutrition, Mount Saint Vincent University, Halifax, NS, Canada
e-mail: Jennifer.Brady@msvu.ca

J. Gingras
Department of Sociology, Ryerson University, Toronto, ON, Canada

© Springer Nature Switzerland AG 2019
J. Coveney, S. Booth (eds.), *Critical Dietetics and Critical Nutrition Studies*,
Food Policy, https://doi.org/10.1007/978-3-030-03113-8_2

Introduction

As its core, Critical Dietetics (CD) is a social justice health movement that seeks to advance justice and equity in all forms.[1] Simply put, axiology describes what is valued or what is considered to be of value. CD axiology comprises the values and core commitments of CD. Herein, we outline the core values and commitments of CD through a discussion of three foundational and interdependent tenets, including a commitment to (1) anti-oppression, (2) critical praxis, and (3) reflexivity. We elaborate on how these tenets give rise to the theoretical, epistemological, methodological, and pedagogical foundations and priorities that inform CD. This paper builds on previously published texts that also outline the core of the CD movement including *Critical Dietetics: A Declaration* (see Gingras and Brady this volume) and *Critical Dietetics: A Discussion Paper* (Gingras et al. 2014).

Our chapter unfolds in three sections. First, we respond to a frequently asked question, "Why theory?" Second, we discuss each of the three tenets noted above. And third, we address another common concern that follows learning about oppression: that sense of overwhelm that can turn learners away from wanting to know more and even immobilize action that may lead to change.

Why Theory?

Theory forms the basis of how we understand complex issues and, through that understanding, take action to generate change. In today's world, we are facing significantly complex issues: economic inequality, racial injustice, sexism, violence, and climate crises to name a few. Many of those reading this chapter will be concerned with and focused on the challenges that reside within the dietetic profession, but we don't take that important work as separate from any broader issues. Despite how overwhelming it may be, as people connected to the food and nutrition profession, we exist interdependently with the world around us. Theory helps forge a path of understanding through these challenges towards meaningful action. Thus, we rely on theory to understand and then act to improve the lives of ourselves and others.

As professors in universities, we hear students say, "Theory is so complicated and boring. Why do I even need to learn it?" We can empathize…to some degree. At the same time, we are fiercely passionate about what theory can do and unabashed about applying theory to challenge our thoughts and, thus, our actions. Like Sears and Cairns (2015), we believe that "Theoretical thinking frames our view of the subject, whether we are conscious of our presuppositions or not" (p. xxi). Perhaps an analogy will be helpful to explain the purpose of theory.

---

[1] For a discussion of definitions of social justice and health equity, see Brady, this volume.

Imagine you are in a house looking outside through a window and you see a visibly distressed woman. The window is angled in such a way that only makes it possible to see this woman. You look beside you at another window, so you move to look through it because you want a different perspective to help make sense of what you see and how you might help this woman. This window is the same size as the first one but angled again to only give you a partial view of the situation. You see a toddler holding someone's hand, but try as you might, the window does not permit you to see who is holding the toddler's hand. Is it the woman? There's another window upstairs. You race to the second floor to figure out what's happening. You see a police officer gesturing with one hand towards something, but you can't see what. You recall there is a third floor to this house, the loft. You are getting desperate to know more. You run upstairs and you see a third person, a man pushing an empty stroller. These windows present us with frames through which to understand what is going on. Different windows or different theories offer different views or different ideas about our world. Our embrace of the view that is offered through each window is influenced by our past experiences and our perceptions. We may notice that one view is preferable since it fits with what we have previously seen (and accepted as true). New views offer new ideas (theories) about what is going on, but we may not accept some views because they may contradict what we have been taught to believe. See how intricate and fascinating theory can be? There are endless points of resonance and disruption when we consider new views of our world as a means to seek meaning. Our understanding of the world reflects our ways of knowing (epistemologies). It is important as professionals to seek as clear a picture as possible of a situation before offering support, so we encourage a trans-theoretical and inter-epistemological approach to practice (multiple theories and multiple ways of knowing). The following tenets of CD, which we offer through our experience with the movement from its inception, aren't to be thought of as rigid boundaries, but more like scaffolding upon which CD can grow and evolve.

Tenets of CD

In this section, we outline three tenets that inform Critical Dietetic axiology, including a commitment to (1) anti-oppression, (2) critical praxis, and (3) reflexivity. It is important to note that these tenets are not meant to stand as a static prescription or formula for CD. The set of tenets presented here, as with CD more generally, are open to expand and change. As the work of Critical Dietitian scholars, practitioners, and students continues, particularly through collaboration from across various disciplines and social locations involved in the struggle for social justice, we expect that these tenets, like CD, will evolve. Nevertheless, the essence of these tenets should be taken as a base requirement of CD that, despite future expansion, must not be undermined. These tenets should be understood as overlapping or interdependent facets that are collectively necessary to the mandate of CD.

Commitment to Anti-oppression

In general terms, being committed to anti-oppression means being oriented through our work, our relationships, and our everyday lives to challenging oppression of all forms including, but not limited to, racism, sexism, classism, colonialism, heteronormativity, homophobia, transphobia, fat bias, ageism, and ableism. More specifically, being committed to anti-oppression requires that we seek out and incorporate into our lives the knowledge and skills needed to effect changes that makes the world a more equitable, just place for all life, as well as for the planet. To effect change we must first understand how oppression and privilege are produced. This tenet, then, comprises a political orientation to equity (fairness) and liberation (freedom) from oppression for all but also a theoretical tool box that allows us to name, pull apart, examine, and ultimately change the very mechanisms by which oppression is produced. The tools in our theoretical tool box are garnered from critical social theory and are indispensable to the knowledge base of CD.

The tools of critical social theory (a particular window) comprise an array of concepts that may be used to describe, explain, and predict how inequities are created, how they organize society, and how they produce oppression. Another important way that the tools, or concepts, of critical social theory are used is in formulating research questions such as, "Why do health inequities persist despite an ever-expanding budget for health care?" The term "critical" in the name critical social theory, and in CD, signals the concern with unearthing how power operates to give rise to and maintain inequities and oppression of all forms. CD adopted the term "critical" purposively to signal its guiding intention to unearth and to end inequity and oppression. To be critical is to be ardently questioning and recognize the urgency of those questions to redress oppression.

Another key concern of critical social theory is related to the ways in which different forms of knowledge are organized hierarchically and how this knowledge hierarchy is intrinsic to the production of oppression. It is imperative for those engaging in anti-oppression efforts, particularly those entrenched in the health sciences, to be mindful of often taken for granted ideas about what counts as knowledge, as well as what is seen as legitimate means of creating knowledge (Gingras 2005). Epistemology is a concept that describes the various ways of understanding what counts as knowledge. Dietetics has traditionally prioritized a positivist epistemology, or positivism (Aphramor and Gingras 2009; DeVault 1995, 1999; Gingras and Brady 2010). Positivism asserts that there exists a singular objective truth to describe any given phenomenon and that the best means of uncovering that objective truth is the scientific method.[2] Knowledge created through the scientific method has dominated the evidence base of dietetics and evidence-based dietetic practice.

---

[2] For a more thorough discussion of epistemology and positivism within dietetics, see Gingras and Brady (2010).

Although we do not wholly reject the scientific method as a means of creating knowledge about the world, a critical orientation rejects the notion that it is even possible to produce knowledge that is objective, value-free, and untouched by human bias. A critical orientation similarly rejects the idea that any one way of creating knowledge about the world is superior to another or is even sufficient. In contrast to positivism, CD is rooted in an interpretivist epistemology, or interpretivism. Interpretivism considers knowledge as inherently subjective and informed by the values, priorities, and worldviews of the individuals, institutions, and wider social, political, and environmental context that guided its creation. An interpretivist epistemology also sees phenomena as being open to multiple means of knowledge creation and interpretation that are equally legitimate. As such, CD draws on post-structuralism and feminist science (two other windows) that hold that there is not one truth that can be generated about any single thing, that multiple truths are possible depending on who is asking and for what purpose, and that knowledge is not apolitical even if it is considered positivist (i.e. value neutral or unbiased). Because humans generate knowledge about phenomena, and humans bring their own beliefs, biases, and assumptions to their knowledge generating processes, the knowledge that humans generate is always subjective. This can be difficult to accept given that we were taught as nutrition students that what we were learning was the truth and there was no point in challenging that truth. For some of us who dared pose questions to challenge nutrition dogma, we risked censure of our critical voice and were sometimes denied access to higher levels of professional autonomy (i.e. we didn't get internships). When we discovered other ways of knowing (e.g. post-structural epistemologies), we learned that food and nutrition epistemology was a more wild, unruly, and unpredictable beast. And, we liked it. And, through CD, we found others that thought similarly.

Critical theoretical concepts are also used to name the means by which oppression is perpetuated at multiple scales and in different ways. At the individual level, oppression may be perpetrated through microaggressions,[3] the subtle everyday intended or unintended acts, such as direct verbal harassment or misrepresentation in the media, that collectively contribute to the social exclusion of oppressed groups (Sue 2010). This concept is important in naming and identifying the additive impact on people's lives of what may otherwise appear to be fleeting and seemingly inconsequential encounters of prejudice, which are actually degrading. At the societal level are institutionalized and structural forms of discrimination that spread oppression in systemic ways. For example, discriminatory hiring practices mean that people of colour, transgender people, women, and fat people are hired and promoted less often and consequently earn less money than those who are white, cis-gender, male-identified, and/or thin (McInturff and Tulloch 2014; Puhl and Heuer 2009). Microaggressions and structural forms of discrimination are mutually reinforcing and together engender oppression. Additionally, social exclusion has a direct

---

[3] Microaggression is a term coined by psychiatrist and Harvard professor Chester M. Pierce in 1970 to describe insults and dismissals he regularly witnessed non-black Americans inflict on African Americans (Wikipedia).

negative impact on individuals' physiological health. The biochemistry of discrimination is a term that describes the way in which social exclusion gets under the skin of oppressed individuals and communities via the physiological chronic stress response that is triggered by that oppression (Butler et al. 2002; Dimsdale et al. 1986; Muenning 2008; Tylka et al. 2014).

Intersectionality is another important concept for understanding and redressing oppression. Crenshaw (1991) coined the term to name the way in which individuals' and communities' experiences of one form of oppression, such as sexism, vary when intersecting with one or more other forms of oppression, such as racism. For example, gender and racial oppression for black women is different than the racial oppression faced by black men and different than gender oppression faced by white women. Black women experience a qualitatively unique form of oppression that is not fully explained when seen as simply the result of additive forms of oppression. Intersectionality is also useful for understanding health inequities. Hankivsky and colleagues have drawn on intersectionality theory to show how health inequities for particular social groups, such as women, are shaped by multiple intersecting social identities, such as race or indigeneity, class, (dis)ability, and so on, that draw out the actual heterogeneity among women as a social category (Hankivsky 2014; Hankivsky and Christofferson 2008; Hankivsky et al. 2010). More recently, others have built on intersectional health research, which has mainly focused on the socio-economic stratification of individuals and communities, to integrate the effects of institutional entities, such as the state, health care, and education, as intersecting components that impact health (Gkiouleka et al. 2018).

Many dietitians are familiar with the social determinants of health: "the circumstances in which people are born, grow up, live, work and age, and the systems put in place to deal with illness" (Mikkonen and Raphael 2010; World Health Organization 2018). However, it is important that we recognize that the social determinants of health are also built in to and reinforced by societal structures such as political and economic systems. Redressing systemic, institutionalized forms of oppression requires that we are conversant with the systems and structures that undergird oppression. Researchers have coined the phrase "structural competence" to call on health professionals to incorporate curriculum about the structural determinants of health into their education and training (Hansen et al. 2018; Metzl and Hansen 2014). Drawing on the work of critical medical anthropologists, Roberts (2009) presents a similar argument in favour of training for health professionals in the structural inequities that result in "structural violence" faced by the poor, women, and people of colour that she serves as a family physician (p. 37). The structural determinants of health acknowledge the influence of institutions (i.e. hospitals, schools), policies, the economy, and infrastructure (i.e. transportation) on the health and capacity to manage individuals and communities. Metzl and colleagues contrast structural competence with the more commonly used framework of cultural competence, which they note merely demands that health professionals know about cultural differences and are conversant in the cultures of individual clients or patients. Conversely, structural competence demands that health professionals appreciate how inequities, specifically health inequities, are produced by social and structural forces that operate beyond individual clients, patients, and practitioners. Others have similarly called on health professionals to recognize and gain competence in the "ecological determinants of health" as the "ultimate determinants of our health" which include "the air we breathe, the water we drink, and the food we eat… [as well as] the materials with which we build our infrastructure and products, and the fuels with which we power them" (Hancock 2017, p. 409). Of related concern are climate change and the consequent environmental degradation that will unfold in the coming years, which will undoubtedly present serious direct health impacts, particularly for oppressed communities, but also indirect health impacts by exacerbating social and health inequities (Alkon and Agyemon 2011).

At a macro-level are the organizing ideologies that inform how we think about health, nutrition, food, and bodies. Critical social theorists have developed important tools with which to name and unpack these ideologies, as well as to examine how these are at play in producing oppression. One example of an organizing ideology is medicalization, which is a concept that describes the way in which everyday issues, experiences, and conditions are redefined as medical problems and brought under the purview of medical management and/or treatment (Conrad 1975). "Obesity"[4] is perhaps the most salient recent example of an aspect of normal human diversity to be medicalized (Aphramor and Gingras 2011a; Austin 1999; Campos et al. 2006). The negative consequences of medicalization extend beyond simple disease mongering. Medicalization may be used to mark a social group as deviant and then bring that group under the control of the "medical gaze" (Foucault 2003), which can worsen oppression and, thus, exacerbate health issues due to stigma and the biochemistry of discrimination.

Another organizing ideology is healthism. Crawford (1980) developed the concept of healthism to describe the growing "preoccupation with personal health as a primary—often *the* primary—focus for the definition and achievement of, well-being" (p. 386, emphasis in original). Crawford (1980) added that health and illness were seen as the result of individual action or inaction—one either worked on being healthy or not—and were taken as proxy indicators of individuals' moral value (p. 380). Related to healthism is another ideology developed by Scrinis (2002, 2008, 2013) called nutritionism. Scrinis described nutritionism as the now dominant paradigm through which we understand and relate to food and wherein food is reduced to little more than vectors for good and bad nutrients. According to Scrinis, the rise of nutritionism has resulted in several negative consequences for our relationship to food and has opened the door for industry to profit from the health halo of their highly processed foods.

It is no coincidence that the rise of healthism and nutritionism coincided with the advancement of another overarching ideology, neoliberalism (Harvey 2005). Neoliberalism has driven much of the social and economic policy that has deepened oppression and further entrenched oppressive systems within social and institutional structures. One example of neoliberalism's impact on health and nutrition is the individual- and commodity-centred way that health, health care, and food are

---

[4] Note that we use scare quote around the term "obesity" to indicate our rejection of the term as an inherently medicalizing and discriminatory word.

now understood. With neoliberalism, the emphasis is on the private sector to provide public services. The government takes the position that they should not interfere with the private sector's primary objective, which is to generate profit. The neoliberal government cuts funding to public services and reduces taxes but continues to subsidize corporations. Together, neoliberalism, medicalization, healthism, and nutritionism have created new and reinforced existing forms of oppression within the realm of health.

Specific examples of the ways in which neoliberalism, medicalization, healthism, and nutritionism have contributed to various forms of oppression abound. One example is the gender binary on which virtually all nutrition recommendations for individuals' caloric intake and nutrient needs are based. The very foundation on which nutrition rests is deeply rooted in the terms of gender-sex-binary, which excludes transgender, gender non-conforming, and gender-queer communities. The strict gender binary leaves little room for conceptualizing the human body as existing outside of the narrowly defined categories for weight, height, sex, and, in some cases, even race. Another example is the ongoing history of surveillance of Indigenous communities using Eurocentric nutrition guidelines (Mosby 2012, 2014; Walters 2012). Milk, in particular, is one food item that has garnered powerful symbolic value as a culturally and nutritionally important food and thereby has been used to medicalize those who traditionally do not or cannot consume dairy due to lactose intolerance. It is no coincidence that those who most often cannot consume dairy foods due to lactose intolerance are Indigenous and other racialized groups (Brady et al. 2016; Dupuis 2002). Yet, a typical neoliberal trade policy has the government propping up the dairy industry through supply management, which limits cross-border competition.

Although critical social theory is an important tool for unearthing the inner workings and consequences of oppression, it is imperative that the voices of those impacted by oppressive systems are at the front and centre of our movements for change. The individuals and communities who are "under threat" by oppressive socially, structurally, and environmentally engendered inequities possess special insight into how oppressive systems work but how those systems impact their everyday lives (McGibbon 2012, p. 32). This also means that those in privileged positions, namely, health professionals who are generally privileged by virtue of their education, position of authority, ethnicity, class, ability, appearance, and gender, must learn when and how to speak out against oppression but also, and perhaps more importantly, how and when to step back and listen to the voices of oppressed communities themselves.

Commitment to Critical Praxis

Although the theoretical tools discussed above are key to illuminating how oppression is produced and the various impacts it has on individuals and groups, theory in and of itself is insufficient to redress inequities. In other words, we are not necessarily advancing social justice just because we count a commitment to anti-oppression among our core values and wield the theoretical tools to unpack it. Hence, this tenet addresses the way in which our principles, and the theories that inform them, must be complemented by practice and action to effect change. In other words, it is necessary to translate our theoretical understanding and political commitment into action. That said, this tenet addresses CD praxis. Paulo Freire (2012) defines praxis as "*reflection and action* directed at the structures to be trans-formed" (p. 32). In other words, praxis, including CD praxis, is the expression of the insights garnered by critical social theory through action for social justice.

The important relationship between theory and dietetic practice is likely not new to many readers of this volume. However, this relationship is traditionally conceived of within the bounds of practice-based research whereby research is carried out within clinical, community, or administrative dietetic practice settings and most often according to the precepts of positivist inquiry (Aphramor and Gingras, 2011b). Drawing on the notion of praxis, CD seeks to expand this relationship between theory and practice beyond practice-based research. CD praxis applies the insights into the working of oppression offered by critical social theory to traditional dietetic practice settings, as well as emerging roles for dietitians as change makers in advocacy and activism. CD praxis urges us to think through what socially just dietetic practice looks like and how dietitians may step into roles as social justice advocates and activists to effect structural, systemic change.

One important area of CD praxis is dietitian education and training. Dietitian education and training is particularly important because they are key sites of professional socialization during which students learn the knowledge and skills required for practice but also assimilate the profession's identity, values, and priorities (MacLellan et al. 2011; MacLellan et al. 2014). Moreover, education is an area of dietetic practice in which anti-oppressive principles may be enacted by educators in the learning process. Socially just pedagogy, that is, *how* and *why* we teach and train dietetic students and interns as educators and preceptors, is as important as what we teach (professional knowledge). Integrating narrative, reflexive, and art-based methods into the classroom can facilitate students' personal connection with their learning.

It is important for dietitian educators, preceptors, and students to remember that *why* we teach is not simply to prepare competent (positivist) dietitians. Our under-graduate and graduate education programmes, as institutions of higher education, are as much readying dietitians for practice, as they are readying citizens to live and participate in the world. Hence, we have a precious opportunity to prepare our future practitioners to not only be competent dietitians but socially responsible citizens that engage in and contribute to their communities and matters of national and global concern. It is not possible to separate one's identity as a competent practitioner and a socially responsible, engaged citizen; nor is such separation is desirable. Rather, we assert that the aim of dietetic education and training should be the preparation of socially responsible dietitian-citizens who draw on their knowledge and authority as nutrition experts to influence changes that enhance social justice.

Dietetic education and training is also an avenue through which dietetic students and interns could be prepared with the knowledge, skills, and confidence to undertake advocacy and activism as aspects of anti-oppressive praxis. Dietetic education and training is vital to enhancing the structural competence of dietetic practitioners. Various health and non-health professions have recognized the crucial role that practitioners play in effecting change for social justice throughout advocacy and have called on educators to better integrate the necessary knowledge- and skilled-based learning that would prepare new practitioners to do so (Braveman and Suarez-Balcazar 2009; Cram 2013; Dharamsi and MacEntee, 2002; Goodman et al. 2004; Hanks 2013; Metzl and Hansen 2014; O'Mahoney Paquin, 2011; Roberts 2009; Swenson 1998). Nevertheless, recent Canadian research suggests that preparation in the skills and knowledge that would enable dietitians to address the structural determinants of health, and social justice more broadly, are seldom included in dietetic undergraduate and graduate programmes (Fraser and Brady forthcoming). What is more, ongoing research by one of the authors (JB) shows that Canadian dietitians report receiving little to no training in this area, and some even leave the profession when their efforts to effect structural level change are thwarted due to lack of training or support from colleagues (Brady 2017; Fraser and Brady forthcoming).

A crucial piece of using one's voice to effect change is being aware of how that voice is positioned in relation to the systems of power, privilege, and oppression that we have discussed above. The next tenet addresses what might be understood as the undergirding and advancing of the first two tenets–reflexivity.

Commitment to Reflexivity

Reflexivity is another tenet at the foundation of CD axiology and is central to CD knowledge and praxis. According to Patton (2015), reflexivity urges us "to be attentive to and conscious of the cultural, political, social, linguistic, and economic origins of one's own perspective and voice as well as the perspective and voices of those one interviews and those to whom one reports. Reflexivity turns mindfulness inward" (p. 70). Patton (2015) adds that reflexivity pushes the more familiar practice of self-reflection further, more "in-depth, experiential, and interpersonal" (p. 69), and involves an "ongoing examination of what I know and how I know it" (p. 70). In other words, reflexivity rouses introspection about one's taken for granted ways of viewing the world but also about how one acquired those ways of viewing the world and how they came to be taken for granted. Examining one's assumptions and the origins of those assumptions obliges one to also question one's positionality in relation to the systems of power, oppression, and privilege that engender hierarchies of knowledge. How one is positioned in relation to systems of power also typically informs where one is placed in relation to the processes of learning and unlearning necessary to understand and redress oppression. Privilege often blinds individuals from seeing the systems that contribute to their unearned position in the world. It is also critical to realize that where one is positioned as privileged, there exist many systems of oppression that have made possible that privilege; thus, reflexivity relies on critical praxis to reinforce one's commitment to anti-oppression.

At first, reflexivity may seem to inspire nothing more than an endless circle of theorization and self-reflection, which runs counter to the commitment to effect social change through action discussed in the second tenet. However, as a facet of CD praxis, reflexivity aims to inspire action in response to the insights unearthed in the process and is key to translating the insights of critical social theory. Reflexivity enables us to see how oppression does not simply operate in the world beyond ourselves, but is present in our unexamined assumptions, and produced and perpetuated through our everyday interactions. Hence, reflexivity is a necessary component of CD praxis that permits individuals to step into their roles as dietetic students, practitioners, advocates, and activists in a way that is mindful of how we are complicit in producing oppression, even when we seek to undo it.

Reflexivity is also not a practice undertaken only by individuals. It is imperative that CD as a collective movement is reflexive about its knowledge base, assumptions, values, and priorities. Moreover, CD must also be reflexive about its position within oppressive systems, such as academia, higher education, and research, as well as health care, and the wider systems of classed, racialized, and gendered knowledge that often infuses thinking about health and nutrition (Biltekoff 2013). Moreover, reflexivity informs how CD as a collective movement understands and approaches its understanding of justice. Justice, and what counts as just, is complex and can be fraught with internal tensions and contradictions. Hence, we draw on DuPuis, Harrison, and Goodman's (2011) notion of "reflexive justice" to acknowledge the ways in which just processes and outcomes are neither perfect nor unchanging. Thus, our collective commitment to anti-oppression and praxis is enlivened by our commitment to undertake the continuous process of examining our cultural, political, social, linguistic, and economic position in the world and, drawing on Patton (2015), asking ourselves "what do we know and how do we know it?"

What does reflexive praxis look like? What does one do when undertaking reflexive praxis? As a commitment to reflexivity, CD reinforces the following activities: open and honest engagement with others; willingness to say "I don't know" and to admit mistakes; authentic examination of feelings, including feelings of overwhelm or guilt; ongoing self-care, particularly for those who work closely within marginalized position(s); active self-compassion coupled with commitment to unpack privilege and strive for equity; relationality, meaning that an open acknowledgement exists that all people are interconnected and interdependent; and an orientation to learning/unlearning, growing, sharpening awareness, and ongoing commitment to all of the above.

At this point in the paper, you may be feeling overwhelmed, especially if this is your first encounter with these tenets. You may be coming to realize that there is so much to learn and to do. We want you to know that everyone experiences this feeling as they confront all that has happened before arriving to this information. You are not alone. And the paradox of natality offers a path forward from this tremendous moment of profound learning and potential transformation.

Paradox of Natality

Natasha Levinson (1997) wrote a compelling article informed by the philosophies of Hannah Arendt in which she described the paradox of natality as that dawning awareness of a particular situation and the simultaneous experience of arriving late to that moment; that much has happened before one became aware of a particular phenomenon. In other words, we all learn about certain issues at varying degrees of time after those issues have originated. Take racism as one example. Before those of us reading this chapter became aware of racism, much harm had been done to racialized people; we arrived to the concept of racism or sexism or homophobia long after these oppressions emerged in society. The sensation of arriving late can leave one feeling stuck by the enormity of the issues or even guilty for the actions of white settlers in the name of colonization, as another example. Alternatively, one might feel like acting to confront racism or settler colonialism even though one was not actually committing those acts; as white settler women, reconciliation has us acknowledging how we have benefitted from those racist acts as well as how we might stand as allies in the effort to redress the harm caused by settler colonialism. For example, in order to redress the legacy of residential schools and advance the process of Canadian reconciliation, the Truth and Reconciliation Commission (2015) made 94 calls to action, including the following: "We call upon medical and nursing schools in Canada to require all students to take a course dealing with Aboriginal health issues, including the history and legacy of residential schools, the *United Nations Declaration on the Rights of Indigenous Peoples*, Treaties and Aboriginal rights, and Indigenous teachings and practices. This will require skills-based training in intercultural competency, conflict resolution, human rights, and anti-racism" (p. 3). We believe this recommendation should be extended to dietetic students.

We wish to emphasize this point about belatedness in the face of learning something new since there may be some of you upon reading this chapter who are experiencing that very thing. You may be asking, "Why didn't I know about this before? Why didn't I learn about this in my dietetic education? How could so much go on around me without me being aware?" We empathize and we want to convey that the important thing is you know now and you can take action. We are a community that offers support (through social media and face-to-face at our conferences) to work through the experience of arriving late. We also believe that since you are a new person coming to these challenging issues, we expect you can bring new life to tackling these problems, hence the paradox of natality; you have arrived new to these issues that have been going on for some time, and you have the power to act in service of making it better for those coming after you. We are in this struggle together.

Furthermore, the burden of overwhelm and guilt can lead to other debilitating situations such as burnout or structural ignorance, where one puts forward a non-critical view even though one knows differently, which only perpetuates systems of oppression. Engaging in structural oppression is to be complicit in reinforcing systems of harm. To the newcomers, we implore you to reach out to those who have authored these chapters for support in negotiating the perils of learning and unlearning. To those who have come to realize their belatedness, and despite the challenges that awareness has brought have chosen to act, we ask that you continue to do so with compassion and courage with a vision to build on the efforts of those who have come before. Additionally, acting with an ethic of care, facilitating growth-fostering relationships, and remembering to celebrate victories however small are also ways to strengthen our movement and our connection.

Conclusion

In this paper, we build on the foundational texts that have already begun to the lay the ground work of CD's knowledge and purpose. With our contribution to that growing body of work, we have sought to address what we are describing as CD axiology—the core values and commitments of CD. We proposed three tenets as one means of conceptualizing CD axiology, including a commitment to (1) anti-oppression, (2) critical praxis, and (3) reflexivity. The core values and commitments of CD as conceptualized by these tents are undergirded by the tools of critical social theory, some of which we have described here, and a dedication to socially just change.

However, we are also sensitive to the challenges that can accompany learning about critical social theory and oppression. Learners often express a sense of confusion and frustration about why they may need or want to learn about critical social theory. Moreover, learners often feel overwhelmed by the complexity and enormity of oppression as it is entrenched in society. That said, our aim in this chapter reaches beyond simply describing the core values of CD. Rather, we seek to mobilize and inspire readers by equipping them with the tools to unpack and redress oppression, as well as with the knowledge that doing so is securely within dietitians' scope of practice. For us, dietitians have a responsibility to undertake learning and action for social change because we have "response ability"; we have the ability to respond to social injustice by virtue of our authority as nutrition and food experts, our education, and other forms of privilege. We hope that this chapter will serve as the beginnings or confirmation of dietitian students and practitioners' acting on their inherent ability to further the commitments of CD that we have presented here.

Assignments

1. Recall the scenario described early on in this paper in which your view of a situation outside is both focused and also limited by the windows of a house. Generate a list of theories that resonate with your current worldview. How did you come to this way of thinking about the world? What experiences shaped how

you see the world around you? What is it about the theories that you chose support and reinforce your worldview? Reflecting on the question asked of you in the preceding chapter, have you changed your way of thinking about the world? Would you have listed the same theories had we asked you this question 5 years ago? Why or why not?

2. Write a short (1–2 pages) reflexive piece in which you discuss the following questions: What do you believe is the role of the dietitian in effecting change related to the issues discussed above? Should dietitians be involved in advocacy and activism? Why or why not? Share your thoughts with a fellow dietitian or classmate. What was their response?

Definition of Keywords and Terms

Anti-oppression	Anti-oppression is an approach or paradigm that is rooted in ending systemic oppression of all kinds, including, but not limited to, racism, sexism classism, homo- and transphobia, sizeism, and so on.
Axiology	Axiology is the study of what is valued, or what is considered to be of value. Critical Dietetic axiology comprises the approaches, knowledges, political commitments, and practices that form the central core of Critical Dietetics.
Critical praxis	Praxis was first defined by scholar-activist Paulo Freire (2012) as "reflection and action directed at the structures to be transformed" (p. 32). For Critical Dietetics, critical praxis comprises the expression of the insights garnered by critical social theory through action for social justice.
Epistemology	Epistemology is a concept that describes the various ways of understanding what counts as knowledge. There are many epistemologies. Mainstream dietetic knowledge and practice are informed by positivist epistemology which understands knowledge creation as the process of uncovering truths about the world through the scientific method. Critical Dietetics is informed by a post-structural epistemology wherein truth is understood as being in constant flux and knowledge creation as requiring multiple, differently situated perspectives, approaches, and methods.
Intersectionality	Intersectionality was coined by feminist legal scholar Kimberle Crenshaw (1991) to describe the ways in which the experience of and social structures supporting one form of oppression vary when intersecting with other forms of oppression.
Microaggression	Microaggressions comprise the subtle everyday intended or unintended acts, such as direct verbal harassment or misrepre-

Reflexivity   sentation in the media, that collectively contribute to the social exclusion of oppressed groups.

Reflexivity describes a practice wherein one is attentive to and reflects critically upon the situated worldview, values, and knowledge of self and others then questioning how those are informed by power, being moved to act to redress inequities, and seeking again to revise worldview, values, and knowledge of self and others based on reflection on action. Reflexivity is not synonymous with reflection given the process does not end with examining worldview, values, and knowledge; this is only the beginning of an iterative (cyclical) process.

How This Chapter Addresses the Critical Dietetic Framework

This chapter addresses all four elements of the Critical Dietetics framework as outlined in this volume. In elaborating the axiological foundations of Critical Dietetics, this chapter provides an in-depth discussion of the values and political commitments that inform the movement including multidisciplinary and trans-theoretical approaches to understanding nutrition, food, health, and people; critical reflexive praxis; knowledge co-creation that values contributions from clients and their families, communities, and service providers; and social just dietetic practice.

References

Alkon AH, Agyemon J (eds) (2011) Cultivating food justice: race, class and sustainability. MIT Press, Cambridge

Aphramor L, Gingras J (2009) That remains to be said: disappeared feminist discourses on fat in dietetic theory and practice. In: Rothblum ED, Solovay S (eds) Fat Studies Reader. New York University Press, New York, pp 97–105

Aphramor L, Gingras J (2011a) Helping people change: promoting politicised practice in the health care professions. In: Rich E, Monaghan LF, Aphramor L (eds) Debating obesity. Palgrave Macmillan, London, pp 192–218

Aphramor L, Gingras J (2011b) Reproducing inequalities: Theories and ethics in dietetics. In: Unnithan-Kumar M, Tremayne S (eds) Fatness and the maternal body: women's experiences of corporeality and the shaping of social policy. Berghan Books, Oxford, pp 205–223

Austin SB (1999) Fat, loathing and public health: the complicity of science in a culture of disordered eating. Cult Med Psychiatry 23(2):245–268

Biltekoff C (2013) Eating right in America: the cultural politics of food and health. Duke University Press, Durham, NC

Brady J (2017) Trading the apron for the white lab coat: a contemporary history of dietetics in Canada, 1954 to 2016. Dissertation, Queen's University

Brady J, Milious V, Ventresca M (2016) Problematizing milk: considering production beyond the food system. In: Anderson CJ, Brady J, Levkoe CZ (eds) Conversations in food studies. University of Manitoba Press, Winnipeg

Braveman B, Suarez-Balcazar Y (2009) Social justice and resource utilization in a community-based organization: a case illustration of the role of the occupational therapist. Am J Occup Ther 63(1):13–23

Butler C, Tull ES, Chambers EC, Taylor J (2002) Internalized racism, body fat distribution, and abnormal fasting glucose among African-Caribbean women in Dominica, West Indies. J Natl Med Assoc 94(3):143–148

Campos P, Saguy A, Ernsberger P, Oliver E, Gaesser G (2006) The epidemiology of overweight and obesity: public health crisis or moral panic? Int J Epidemiol 35(1):55–60

Conrad P (1975) The discovery of hyperkinesis: notes on the medicalization of deviant behaviour. Soc Probl 23(1):12–21

Cram B (2013) University continuing education units: agents for social change? Can J Univ Contin Educ 31(1)

Crawford R (1980) Healthism and the medicalization of everyday life. Int J Health Serv 10(3):365–388. https://doi.org/10.2190/3H2H-3XJN-3KAY-G9NY

Crenshaw K (1991) Mapping the margins: intersectionality, identity politics, and violence against women of color. Stan L Rev 43(6):1241–1299

DeVault M (1995) Between science and food: nutrition professionals in the health-care hierarchy. In: Kronenfeld JJ (ed) Research in the sociology of health care. JAI Press, Inc, Greenwich, CT, pp 287–312

DeVault M (1999) Whose science of food and health? Narratives of profession and activism from public-health nutrition. In: Clarke AE, Olesen VL (eds) Revisioning women, health, and healing: feminist, cultural, and technoscience perspectives. Routledge, New York, pp 166–186

Dharamsi S, MacEntee MI (2002) Dentistry and distributive justice. Soc Sci Med 55(2):323–329

Dimsdale JE, Pierce C, Schoenfeld D, Brown A, Zusman R, Graham R (1986) Suppressed anger and blood pressure: the effects of race, sex, social class, obesity, and age. Psychosom Med 48(6):430–436

Dupuis M (2002) Nature's perfect food: how milk became America's drink. NYU Press, New York

DuPuis M, Harrison JL, Goodman D (2011.) Just food?) In: Alkon AH, Agyeman J (eds) Cultivating food justice: race, class, and sustainability. MIT Press, Cambridge, MA, pp 283–308

Foucault M (2003) The birth of the clinic. Taylor and Francis, Florence

Fraser K, Brady J (forthcoming) Exploring social justice advocacy in dietetic education: a content analysis. Can J Diet Pract Res

Freire P (2012) Pedagogy of the oppressed, 30th edn. Bloomsberry Academic, New York

Gingras J (2005) Evoking trust in the nutrition counselor: why should we be trusted? J Agric Environ Ethics 18(1):57–74

Gingras J, Brady J (2010) To be other: relational consequences of dietitians feeding bodily difference. Rad Psychol 8(1)

Gingras J, Asada Y, Fox A, Coveney J, Berenbaum S, Aphramor L (2014) Critical dietetics: a discussion paper. J Crit Diet 2(1):2–12

Gkiouleka A, Huijts T, Beckfield J, Bambra C (2018) Understanding the micro and macro politics of health: inequalities, intersectionality & institutions. Soc Sci Med 200:92–98

Hancock T (2017) Population health promotion in the anthropocene. In: Rootman I, Pederson A, Frohlich KL, Dupere S (eds) Health promotion in Canada: new perspectives on theory, practice, policy, and research. Canadian Scholars Press, Toronto, pp 408–433

Hankivsky O (2014) Intersectionality 101. The Institute for Intersectionality Research and Policy. Available via http://vawforum-cwr.ca/sites/default/files/attachments/intersectionallity_101.pdf. 24 April 2018

Hankivsky O, Christofferson A (2008) Intersectionality and the determinants of health: a Canadian perspective. Crit Public Health 18(3):271–283

Hankivsky O, Reid C, Cormier R, Varcoe C, Clark N, Benoit C, Brotman S (2010) Exploring the promises of intersectionality for advancing women's health research. Int J Equity Health 9(5):1–15

Hanks RG (2013) Social advocacy: a call for nursing action. Pastoral Psychol 62:163–173

Hansen H, Braslow J, Rohrbaugh RM (2018) From cultural to structural competency: training psychiatry residents to act on social determinants of health and institutional racism. JAMA Psychiat 75(2):117–118

Harvey D (2005) A brief history of neoliberalism. Oxford University Press, New York

Goodman LA, Liang B, Helms JE, Latta RE, Sparks E, Weintraub SR (2004) Training counseling psychologists as social justice agents: feminist and multicultural principles in action. Couns Psychol 32(6):793–836

Levinson N (1997) Teaching in the midst of belatedness: the paradox of natality in Hannah Arendt's educational thought. Educ Theory 47(4):435–451

MacLellan D, Lordly D, Gingras J (2011) Professional socialization in dietetics: a review of the literature. Can J Diet Pract Res 72(1):37–42

MacLellan D, Lordly D, Gingras J (2014) On beginning to become dietitians. J Crit Diet 2(1):13–20

McGibbon EA (2012) People under threat: health outcomes and oppression. In: McGibbon EA (ed) Oppression: a social determinant of health. Fernwood Publishing, Halifax, NS

McInturff K, Tulloch P (2014) Narrowing the Gap: The Difference that Public Sector Wages Make. Canadian Centre for Policy Alternatives. Available via https://www.policyalternatives.ca/sites/default/files/uploads/publications/National%20Office/2014/10/Narrowing_the_Gap.pdf. Accessed 18 April 2018

Metzl JM, Hansen H (2014) Structural competency: theorizing a new medical engagement with stigma and inequality. Soc Sci Med 103:126–133

Mikkonen J, Raphael D (2010) Social determinants of health: The Canadian facts. Available via http://thecanadianfacts.org. Accessed 24 April 2018

Mosby I (2014) Food will win the war: the politics, culture, and science of food on Canada's home front. UBC Press, Vancouver

Mosby I (2012) Making and breaking Canada's food rules: science, the state, and the government of nutrition. In: Iacovetta F, Korinek VJ, Epp M (eds) Edible histories, cultural politics: towards a Canadian food history. University of Toronto Press, Toronto, pp 409–432

Muenning P (2008) The body politic: the relationship between stigma and obesity-associated disease. BMC Pub Health 8:128–137

O'Mahoney Paquin S (2011) Social justice advocacy in nursing: what is it? How do we get there? Creat Nurs 17(2):63–67

Patton MQ (2015) Qualitative research & evaluation methods, 4th edn. Sage, Los Angeles, CA

Puhl RM, Heuer CA (2009) The stigma of obesity: a review and update. Obesity 17(5):941–964

Roberts JH (2009) Structural violence and emotional health: a message from Easington, a former mining community in Northern England. Anthropol Med 16(1):37–48

Scrinis G (2002) Sorry Marge. Meanjin 61(4):108–110

Scrinis G (2008) On the ideology of nutritionism. Gastronomica 8(1):39–48

Scrinis G (2013) Nutritionism: the science and politics of dietary advice. Columbia University Press, New York

Sears A, Cairns J (2015) A good book, in theory: making sense through inquiry, 3rd edn. University of Toronto Press, Toronto, ON

Sue DW (2010) Microaggressions in everyday life: race, gender, and sexual orientation. John Wiley & Sons, New Jersey, NY

Swenson CR (1998) Clinical social work's contribution: a social justice perspective. Soc Work 43(6):527–537

Tylka TL, Annunziato RA, Burgard D, Danielsdottir S, Shuman E, Davis C, Calogero RM (2014) The weight-inclusive versus weight-normative approach to health: evaluating the evidence for prioritizing well-being over weight loss. J Obesity 2014:1. https://doi.org/10.1155/2014/983495

Walters K (2012) A national priority: nutrition Canada's survey and the disciplining of aboriginal bodies, 1964-1975. In: Iacovetta F, Korinek VJ, Epp M (eds) Edible histories, cultural politics: towards a Canadian food history. University of Toronto Press, Toronto, pp 433–451

World Health Organization (2018) Social determinants of health: Key concepts. Available from http://www.who.int/social_determinants/thecommission/finalreport/key_concepts/en/index.html. Accessed 16 April 2018

Further Reading and Resources

Beautiful Rising

An international network of advocates, activists, and change makers. The website offers stories of change-making campaigns as well as reading materials, tools, and resources for those interested in undertaking creative action for social change

https://beautifulrising.org

McIntosh P (1988) White privilege and male privilege: a personal account of coming to see correspondences through work in women's studies. Working Paper 189 (1988), Wellesley Centers for Women, Wellesley College, MA, 02481. Retrieved April 5 2018 from https://national-seedproject.org/images/documents/White_Privilege_and_Male_Privilege_Personal_Account-Peggy_McIntosh.pdf

Lee B, Sammon S, Dumbrill GC (2014) Glossary of terms for anti-oppressive policy and practice. Commonact Press, Toronto

Truth and Reconciliation Commission of Canada (2015) Truth and Reconciliation Commission of Canada: Calls to Action. Retrieved April 5 2018 from http://www.trc.ca/websites/trcinstitution/File/2015/Findings/Calls_to_Action_English2.pdf

Chapter 3
Swimming Upstream: Bringing Critical Dietetics into Conventional Practice

Debbie MacLellan

Aim of Chapter and Learning Outcomes

The aim of this chapter is to describe how dietitians are socialized in the early years of practice and the challenges dietitians face in incorporating the tenets of critical dietetics into their day-to-day practice.

At the end of this chapter, readers will:

(i) Describe the shift from our roots in the humanistic, holistic and social justice approaches characteristic of home economics towards a more biomedical model of practice.
(ii) Understand how the hierarchy of practice and what we count as evidence has influenced the way in which power has shifted within the dietetic profession.
(iii) Understand how dietitians are socialized into the profession.
(iv) Identify the gaps in the research related to socialization and identity formation in the dietetic profession and the relationship between these concepts and the Critical Dietetics Framework.

Summary

Critical dietetics began with a small group of like-minded professionals dissatisfied by the current state of the dietetic profession around the world and who were seeking change. We wanted to redefine the profession, to expand our understanding of what it means to be a dietitian and to move beyond the biomedical model of practice. Although, in recent years, our education system has expanded to consider

D. MacLellan, PhD (✉)
University of Canada, New Cairo, Egypt
e-mail: maclellan@upei.ca

© Springer Nature Switzerland AG 2019
J. Coveney, S. Booth (eds.), *Critical Dietetics and Critical Nutrition Studies*,
Food Policy, https://doi.org/10.1007/978-3-030-03113-8_3

non-nutritional determinants of health, we know from recent research that new dietitians are not prepared for the relational and "messy" aspects of our work. Many enter the profession wanting to help people by telling them what to eat, something that we have known for many years does not create lasting behaviour change. When they find that their clients present to them with multiple medical problems, lack of food security, mental illness and other issues related to the social determinants of health, many burn out and may leave the profession. In this chapter I will explore how dietitians are socialized in the early years of practice and then discuss how we can start to "swim upstream" to work towards a new way of way of practising that incorporates the tenets of critical dietetics.

Introduction

I have been a dietetic educator in Canada for almost 30 years, and during that time I have seen some changes, mainly in the way the dietetic profession is regulated and the competencies and knowledge statements that have been developed to guide the structure of our dietetic education programmes. In addition, we have adopted technology as our primary way of communicating with one another and have strongly endorsed evidence-based practice as the basis of everything we do as dietitians. Unfortunately this has meant a shift away from our roots and towards a "troubling divide between food and nutrition" (Sharp 2012).

Prior to the eighteenth century, women were held in high esteem as healers through the use of herbs, spices and other foods in the use of medicinal cookery (Liquori 2001). However, when medical sciences started to emerge as a reputable profession, women were relegated to domestic work to allow room for male physicians to minister to the sick. In the late nineteenth century, women were able to establish themselves as professional home economists, through their knowledge of nutrition, sanitation and childrearing, and university programmes were implemented worldwide; however, it proved impossible to improve the reputation of the home economics profession. It was still seen as an extension of "women's work" in the home, and gradually the university programmes, at least in North America, changed their names and eliminated the applied social science components of home economics in order to compete with more positivist professions, particularly medicine (Liquori 2001; Sharp 2012).

The dietetic profession, in particular, has worked hard over the years to move away from our home economics roots in an attempt to improve our status among healthcare professionals and to establish ourselves as valued members of the healthcare team. In doing so we adopted a biomedical model of practice and lost the more humanistic, holistic and social justice approaches that were characteristic of the home economics profession. We also, perhaps unknowingly, created a hierarchy within the profession "…that views nutrition as the premium entrée and food in all of its experiential dimensions as the day-old-bread" (Power 2011). We continue to see that hierarchy among different aspects of the profession as well. Dietitians who work in the areas of food service and the food industry are not as highly respected as clinical dietitians. We also see a hierarchy in terms of the evidence that we deem high quality (randomized controlled trials) versus qualitative research and clinical judgement which are considered to be of lesser quality. At the heart of these hierarchies lies the issue of power. As Dr. Elaine Power (2011) stated:

> In our lived world of hierarchical power relations, some people win, some people lose, some people speak and are heard, others speak but no one hears; some knowledge is valid other knowledge is not. (p. 13)

Dietitians tend to work in subordinate positions within the healthcare system and thus have less power than those at the top of the hierarchy (physicians, surgeons, etc.). In order to gain power, we have had to incorporate the positivist, reductionist model of medical knowledge into our education and practice and position ourselves as nutrition experts, ignoring "the embodied food knowledge of our patients and clients" (Power 2011, p. 13).

In the previous chapter, Lordly and colleagues explored the changes that need to be made in dietetic education and training in order to facilitate a cultural shift that allows for a critical dietetic approach to practice. In this chapter, I will extend that thinking to explore how dietitians are socialized in the early years of practice and how we can start to "swim upstream" to work towards a new way of practising that incorporates the tenets of critical dietetics.

Professional Socialization and Identity Formation in Dietetics

There is very little research on how dietitians are socialized into the profession and form an identity as a dietitian. Unlike other health professionals who enter their programmes in a cohort model and are being socialized into their professions from the day they start their education, students who want to be dietitians have to start in an accredited nutrition programme but may or may not be accepted into the practicum portion of dietetic education and therefore may or may not become a dietitian. Thus, unlike other allied health professions, such as nursing, physiotherapy and occupational therapy, research has shown that dietetic students focus on becoming an intern during their undergraduate education rather than starting to develop an identity as a dietitian (MacLellan et al. 2011). They are forced to compete with their peers to obtain an internship placement which creates a "culture of competition" that limits students' engagement in their learning, has implications for their health and wellbeing and encourages a "bare minimum" approach to learning (Lordly and MacLellan 2008). This has negative implications for how one becomes a dietitian and can lead to feelings of inadequacy and not being prepared for the realities of practice.

In 2013, I was involved in a research project with several Canadian colleagues to explore the processes of professional socialization and identity development in dietitians in the early stage of their careers (3 years or less). This research, which was presented as vignettes or composite stories, uncovered several issues that made those early years problematic (MacLellan et al. 2013). Our findings indicated the new dietitians struggle to develop their dietitian identity and find the transition from dietetic intern to dietitian challenging. In particular, they feel unprepared for the relational and practice realities of the workplace.

Professional socialization is a process of learning the formal knowledge, skills and rules associated with becoming a professional (Goldenberg and Iwasiw 1993). It is the "process by which people selectively acquire the values and attitudes, the interests, skills and knowledge – in short, the culture – current in groups of which they are, or seek to become, a member" (Clouder 2003, p. 213). This process contributes to the development of a professional identity; however, there is a paucity of research on the culture of the dietetic profession. Lordly (2016) explored one aspect of the socialization and acculturation processes in her research on what counts as dietetic knowledge. Her findings suggest that:

> Dietitians may unknowingly be operating from within an ideological frame that perpetuates the homogenation and the hierarchization of dietetic knowledge.
> A knowledge status quo is created as discussions about dietetic knowledge are captured within an ideological circle and perpetuated by the textual representation of official dietetic knowledge that is activated by dietetic practitioners. (p. 43)

Lordly (2016) also talks about the "standardized dietitian" who is created through our regulated education processes (p. 44). These terms (homogenation, hierarchization and standardized) suggest that our profession values certain types of knowledge over others and that through the processes of selecting and educating dietetic interns, we are cloning competent and good dietitians who resemble ourselves as dietetic educators. Guthman (2014) voiced similar concerns when she wrote: "While not explicitly stated in the declaration [Critical Dietetics: A Declaration, 2009), much of the critical dietetics movement has been a reaction to what geographers Hayes-Conroy and Hayes-Conroy (2013) have dubbed "hegemonic nutrition". Further Guthman (2014) states:

> By hegemonic nutrition, they refer to a set of discourses and practices that (a) assume that food, and thus the food-body relationship, can be standardized to a one size fits all approach; (b) assume that nourishment can be reduced to and then meted out through universal metrics of calories, nutrients and so forth, and (c) neglect cultural, social and historical contexts in both knowledge of good food and enjoyment of it. (p. 1)

If this is true, and my experience as a dietetic educator leads me to believe that it is, how can we begin to create space for new ways of knowing and "...expand traditional theoretical frameworks beyond conventional ways of thought and practice" (Gingras et al. (2014).

Swimming Upstream: "Beyond the Stable State"[1]

In 1971, Donald Schon wrote:

---

[1] Schon, D. (1971) Beyond the Stable State: Public and private learning in a changing society.

Belief in the stable state is belief in the unchangeability, the constancy of central aspects of our lives, or belief that we can attain such a constancy. Belief in the stable state is strong within us. We institutionalize it in every social domain.

We do this in spite of our talk about change, our apparent acceptance of change and our approval of dynamism.....Moreover, talk about change is as often as not a substitute for engaging in it. (p. 9)

Although this was written almost 50 years ago, I think that this belief in the stable state is still pervasive in the dietetic profession. Despite the fact that mentioned, changes have been made to ensure that our graduates are safe to practice and there have been improvements in technology and how we communicate with one another. However, I don't believe that the way we educate and socialize new dietitians into the profession or the way we educate and counsel our clients has changed significantly. If anything, we have taken several steps backwards in Canada with the implementation of the Integrated Competencies for Dietetic Education and Practice which has rendered dietetic education into a series of tasks that must be completed. Although some may argue that there are many dietitians now working in nontraditional areas, I would say that dietetics continues to be a very traditional profession; most dietitians do not embrace change very easily. As a result, the idea of shifting to a new way of thinking and making a commitment to the tenets of critical dietetics seems difficult, if not impossible. However, if we are to survive and thrive as a profession in the twenty-first century, we must find ways to do so.

Over 10 years ago, Sue McGregor (2006) wrote about transformative practice and adopting a critical science approach to the home economics profession. I believe that we can learn a lot from her discussion of these issues and her suggestions regarding paradigm shifts and the need for transformative leadership. She begins her book by saying that "This entire book is predicated on the assumption that a profession has to be open to a paradigm shift" (p. 1). She then proceeds to state that her understanding of a paradigm shift "...refers to a set of experiences, beliefs, values, and assumptions that profoundly affect the way a person perceives reality and responds to that perception. When this personal belief system changes, the person experiences a paradigm shift" (p. 1).

Most, if not all, of us involved in the 2008 research workshop "Beyond Nutritionism: Rescuing Dietetics Through Critical Dialogue" had already begun this change in our belief system regarding mainstream dietetics. But it was that workshop that solidified the need for change "...to define, deconstruct and re-create the future of our profession together" (Gingras et al. 2014, p. 2). Since that time we have held several international conferences where we have invited researchers and professionals from many different areas, and slowly the movement has been gaining momentum. But to make a significant difference, and for an entire profession to undergo a paradigm shift, a state of crisis must emerge "...because too many things are happen[ing] that cannot be explained using the assumptions of the dominant paradigm. Under these circumstances, people become much more willing to explore ideas that were once unthinkable" (McGregor 2006, p. 1). In Canada, at least, I

London: Temple Smith.

think that crisis has begun. Fewer dietitians are joining our national organization, Dietitians of Canada, and many are not renewing after years of membership. New Facebook groups have emerged that allow dietitians to vent their frustrations regarding the way that they are "allowed" to practise which suggests to me that the status quo, professional association and most definitely the regulatory bodies are not providing some members with what they are looking for.

Recently, I spoke to a former student of mine, who became a dietitian about 5 years ago but has not renewed her licence this year. She told me that she is no longer registered because of the rigidity of the places she had worked, environments that did not allow her to practice in a holistic and client-centred way (personal communication, May 2018). When asked if she knew of others who were like minded, she stated clearly and unequivocally that there were many of her classmates who were also disappointed and who were seeking other ways to assist clients live healthier lives without handing them a pamphlet.

So what needs to be done to ramp up our efforts to incorporate the tenets of critical dietetics into dietetic practice? I believe that the answer lies primarily in how we educate and train future dietitians as discussed in the previous chapter. We need a critical mass of people who are willing to challenge the status quo and to advocate "…for more social, political and economic understandings of health into our practice" (Gingras et al. 2014, p. 3). However, since this chapter is about dietitians already in practice, I would suggest the following actions:

(a) A small group of dietitians who are committed to the tenets of critical dietetics have started working on formalizing the organization and spreading the word through informal and formal discussions/presentations with colleagues around the world. Previously, we had difficulty in spreading the word about critical dietetics because our national journals were hesitant to publish any work that suggested we were being "critical" of our profession. Further, and even more disturbing, was a comment that a colleague received from a reviewer who did not consider any topics related to critical dietetics as relevant to our practice. I have seen some change in Canada in regard to publishing research previously considered "not relevant to dietetic practice", but we still have a long way to go there. Fortunately we have the *Journal of Critical Dietetics* that offers researchers from a wide variety of areas an arena to discuss issues that challenge the boundaries of mainstream dietetics. We have created a committee to spread the work of the journal among more people and have been tasked to spread the word about the work we are publishing and encouraging colleagues to start using this research in their journal clubs and become members of Critical Dietetics. Ideally my hope is that Dietitians of Canada and Critical Dietetics become partners or one organization that embraces differing viewpoints and differing ways of knowing.

(b) The word "critical" often evokes a feeling of discomfort and sometimes fear among dietetic professionals. They may feel that this implies that we are not doing a good job which might further undermine our perceived value among the healthcare team. Again, we need to alleviate these concerns and present Critical

Dietetics as a movement that values other forms of knowledge and research methods (beyond the technical, rational approach and the reliance on the clinical trial). In doing so, "…we create the possibility of gaining a better understanding of how to best respond to nutrition-related issues more comprehensively" (Gingras et al. 2014, p. 4). This should excite those dietitians who are dissatisfied with the status quo and help to build the critical mass of people we need to spread the word.

(c) We need to recognize that there are workplace barriers that will need to be addressed and that likely will not be easy or quick to overcome. Again, I believe that as more and more dietitians are educated and exposed to how critical dietetics can improve their practice and offer a better way to help our clients to be active participants in their care, we will be able to use our collective voice to address the barriers.

(d) One of the key elements of professional practice in healthcare today is the concept of evidence-based practice. In Canada, Dietitians of Canada has spent a lot of resources on the development of evidence-based guidelines and the grading of that evidence to enable dietitians to base their decisions on primarily quantitative scientific research. The PEN (Practice-based Evidence in Nutrition) database is now being used by several countries around the world by dietitians who want to provide their clients with treatment interventions based on sound scientific evidence. PEN relies heavily on a hierarchy of evidence that places clinical judgement and qualitative research (considered soft evidence) at the bottom of that hierarchy and the "gold standard" (the double-blind, placebo-controlled, clinical trial, considered hard evidence) at the top. Thus, the art of dietetic practice "…which is essential to developing clinical expertise and judgement is not adequately reflected in the research literature and the term evidence-based practice has become synonymous with scientific research evidence" (Williams and Paterson 2009, p. 689). These authors also found that professional artistry is crucial to the development of therapeutic relationships with their clients and that the satisfaction that practitioners derived from professional artistry led to greater job satisfaction and a greater valuing of the professional (Williams and Paterson 2009, p. 714). Schön's seminal 1983 book, *The Reflective Practitioner*, challenged practitioners to reconsider the role of technical knowledge versus "artistry" in developing professional excellence. It is time to bring back the artistry of practice that was lost in the movement away from Home Economics to dietetic programmes focussed on nutritional science. This has already begun in many places around the world. In Canada, several of my colleagues are incorporating arts-based projects into their dietetic courses. Further, many other health professionals have started to use art as a way of expressing their feelings of hope, despair, loss, etc. which has enriched their practice and has demonstrated in a way that words cannot express, the challenges associated with being a helping professional.

(e) In this social media age, there are many dietitians promoting their businesses and sometimes even doing business on the internet. A critical dietetics blog might be one way to expand our reach and encourage people (perhaps more than just dietitians) to start thinking differently about how they practise.

(f) Last, but certainly not least, is the need to create a culture where reflexivity is the norm in our practice and not just during dietetic education. "Critical health professions have identified reflexive practice as a means to avoid the "detached, objective technician of the scientist-practitioner model into a reflective, engaged and invested social actor" (Gingras et al. 2014, p. 6).

Conclusion

According to Chapman (2011), "Critical dietetics means addressing these 'upstream' issues" (p. 3) and ",,,,, presents our profession with an opportunity to broaden our perspective, and refocus on the issues, opportunities, strategies that are needed to make the shift to a culture that values and supports 'eating well' with all of the richness that food and eating entail" (p. 3).

Why is it worth swimming upstream to incorporate critical dietetics with mainstream dietetics? I fear that the rising discontent that I have observed brewing over the last couple of years may mean the demise of our professional association, similar to what happened to the Canadian Home Economics Association (CHEA). I'm not sure if things are that dire in other parts of the world, but having lived through the demise of CHEA, I can see the writing on the wall in Canada. If we don't change the way we practice, we will not be able to keep up with the increasingly difficult problems that our clients face and we will continue to lose new practitioners as they struggle to deal with the realities of practice. Those of us who have been involved in the critical dietetic movement since its inception know that conventional wisdom, rooted in the biosciences, must be balanced with other ways of knowing. This will allow us to have a deeper understanding of the multiplicity of problems we are being called upon to address. In 2005, Berenbaum challenged us to think more creatively, to take risk and to challenge the status quo. It is time to take up the challenge on a broader scale, to find ways to overcome the barriers to change, to engage in reflexive practice and to conduct research that directly serves the communities studied "…by connecting lived experience with social environments and structures" (Travers 1997).

Assignments

1. Provide participants with a copy of the discussion paper on critical dietetics (Gingras et al. (2014) Critical dietetics: A discussion paper. Journal of Critical Dietetics 2(1). Ask them to write a reflective response to the following question: Using the ideas proposed in this paper, reflect on how different your work might be if these ideas were put into practice.

2. Identify any barriers to the implementation of the Critical Dietetics Framework into mainstream dietetic practice. Discuss how those barriers might be overcome.
3. In groups of 5, discuss the questions you still have about critical dietetics after reading this chapter and how we might incorporate those ideas into conventional practice.
4. What does reflexive practice mean to you? How might you incorporate this practice into your daily work life as a dietitian?
5. Provide participants with a copy of the discussion paper on critical dietetics (Gingras et al. (2014) Critical dietetics: A discussion paper. Journal of Critical Dietetics 2(1): 2–12. Ask them to write a response to the following question: In this paper, the authors only focus on one area of practice to provide examples of how dietitians can incorporate the tenets of critical dietetics into nutrition education. Using your own area of practice, reflect on things that you could do in your own area of influence to incorporate critical dietetic principles into dietetic practice.
6. In groups of 5, discuss the questions you still have about critical dietetics after reading Gingras et al.'s paper and how we might incorporate those ideas into conventional practice.

Definition of Keywords and Terms

Professional identity	This is a concept that describes how we perceive ourselves as professionals and how we communicate that to others.
Professional socialization	Socialization is the process by which individuals acquire the identity of a professional. This process involves the learning of the values norms behaviours and social skills associated with their profession
Reflexivity	When one is practising reflexivity, she is going beyond reflecting on an experience and how she can improve practice as a result. Reflexivity involves exploring one's feelings, motives and reactions to a situation and how this influences her thinking about that situation.
Standardised dietitian	The process by which professional education and professional practices inculcate a particular standardized subjectivity.
Transformative practice	This is a way of practising that results in beneficial change.

How This Chapter Addresses the Critical Dietetics Framework

This chapter addresses the Critical Dietetics Framework in its commitment to reflexive practice and to the co-production of knowledge.

References

Berenbaum S (2005) Imagination nourishes dietetic practice: 2005 Ryley-Jeffs Memorial Lecture. Can J Diet Prac Res 66:193–196

Clouder L (2003) Becoming professional: exploring the complexities of professional socialization in health and social care. Learn Health Soc Care 2:213–222

Chapman G (2011) What 'critical dietetics' means to me. J Crit Diet 1:3

Gingras J, Asada Y, Fox A, Coveney J, Berenbaum S, Aphramor L (2014) Critical dietetics: A discussion paper. J Crit Diet 2:2–12

Goldenberg D, Iwasiw D (1993) Professional socialization of nursing students as an outcome of a senior clinical preceptorship experience. Nurse Educ Today 13:3–15

Guthman J (2014) Introducing critical nutrition: a special issue on dietary advice and its discontents. Gastronomica 13:1–4

Hayes-Conroy A, Hayes-Conroy J (eds) (2013) Doing nutrition differently: critical approaches to diet and dietary intervention. Ashgate, Surrey

Liquori T (2001) Food matters: changing dimensions of science and practice in the nutrition profession. J Nutr Educ 33:234–246

Lordly D (2016) The trusted expert as an ideological code: the socialization of dietetic knowledge. J Crit Diet 3:43–49

Lordly D, MacLellan D (2008) Acknowledging and adapting to dietetic students' changing needs. Can J Diet Pract Res 69:126–130

MacLellan D, Lordly D, Gingras J (2011) Professional socialization: an integrative review of the literature and implications for dietetic education. Can J Diet Prac Res 72:37–42

MacLellan D, Gingras J, Lordly D, Brady J (2013) On beginning to become dietitians. J Crit Diet 2:26–32

McGregor S (2006) Transformative practice: new pathways to leadership. Kappa Omicron Nu Honor Society, East Lansing

Power E (2011) Critical dietetics: understanding power relations & promoting food as nourishment. J Crit Diet 1:13

Sharp A (2012) A recipe for obselesence: the troubling divide between food and nutrition (part one). J Crit Diet 1:3.

Travers K (1997) Reducing inequities through participatory research and community engagement. Health Educ Behav 24:344–356

Williams S, Paterson M (2009) A phenomenological study of the art of occupational therapy. Qual Report 14:689–718

Chapter 4
Awakening the Possibilities: An Exploration of Critical Nutrition and Dietetic Training and Education

Daphne Lordly, Elin Lövestam, and Jillian Ruhl

Aim and Learning Outcomes

The aim of this chapter is to introduce readers to nutrition and dietetic training and education practices or processes that can limit or extend our capacity to engage in more critically informed ways of knowing.

At the end of this chapter, readers will:

(i) Reflect upon their own educational experiences, and express in what ways their learnings were shaped.
(ii) Articulate the elements of the safe space concept, and recognize how the learning environment can influence inclusion, relational work, the diversity of conversation and the cocreation of more complete knowledge and learning.
(iii) Evaluate how they themselves are implicated in the practices and processes that are situated within dominant values and ways of knowing.

Summary

Students need to be afforded with an education of systemic problems in order to deal with modern-day world issues connected to food, health and people. Critical dietetics education bridges the gap that separates conventional positivist

D. Lordly (✉) · J. Ruhl
Department of Applied Human Nutrition, Mount Saint Vincent University,
Halifax, NS, Canada
e-mail: Daphne.Lordly@msvu.ca

E. Lövestam
Department of Food Studies, Nutrition and Dietetics Uppsala University, Uppsala, Sweden

© Springer Nature Switzerland AG 2019   43
J. Coveney, S. Booth (eds.), *Critical Dietetics and Critical Nutrition Studies*,
Food Policy, https://doi.org/10.1007/978-3-030-03113-8_4

perspectives in food and nutrition from studies in the humanities and natural and social sciences. Without a background and learned appreciation of multidisciplinary and trans-theoretical approaches, nutritional practices cannot be far-reaching and sustainable. This chapter focuses on how academic institutions dictate knowledge through structured practices that may limit relational work and limit the possibilities offer by a more critical perspective. This chapter illuminates the importance of being reflexive in work with and among colleagues in order to shape future practices in dietetics and nutrition. This chapter provides a unique perspective on how to cocreate knowledge in the classroom by challenging traditional hierarchical education models. The educational environment is a crucial factor in the development of students' identities, confidence and professionalism. By facilitating a space for exposing authenticity and vulnerability, students may be better equipped for building genuine relationships with clients and colleagues and finding their voice for key decision-making. Respecting student voice and acknowledging the importance of diverse experience foster perspective-taking and sensitivity to multidimensional problems. Building upon students' diverse histories as a means to become change agents is necessary for training an influential workforce.

Beginning Assignment

Before this next chapter, take a minute to reflect on your educational experience. Were there times inside or outside the classroom when you felt engaged, inspired, disappointed or ashamed? What was it about those times that made you feel that way? What was the classroom layout like? What type of teaching activities or engagement techniques did the professor use? Was there a particular individual or group assignment that resonated with you? Using a separate sheet of paper or the mind map outlined below, jot down words, phrases or brief descriptions about the specific factors you remember particularly well. Some themes you may want to reflect on include the course subject matter, the professor, the students, the classroom, assignments/projects, field trips/labs, guest speakers, volunteer work, school-life-work balance, student societies and family. Looking at your mind map, why do you think these elements stood out for you? How will these memorable aspects of your educational experience shape your future practice?

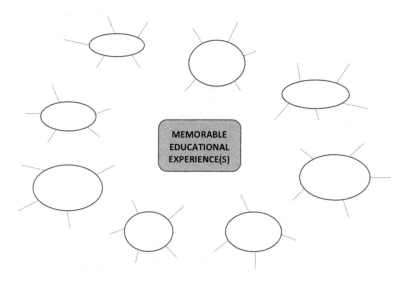

As you read through the following experiences and dialogue, reflect on how your experiences in your mind map intersect or diverge with that of the authors.

Section 1: Creating a Feeling of Safeness, a Safe Space

Can you share an educational experience that resonated with you, assisted in your growth as a student or an educator?

Teacher Quote

I [Daphne] learn so much from my students. Much of my personal growth as an educator can be attributed to them. For me the classroom is *our* space – not my space. I am an academic, but my career trajectory was not one of a typical academic. It was not a Bachelor's, a Master's and then a Doctoral degree. I worked as a dietitian in a hospital for many years and started my Master's on a part-time basis as a result of a job change. I had moved to a different province and was hired as a university Dietetic Internship Coordinator. I also began teaching part-time. I really enjoyed working with students. The Coordinator position was eventually converted to a faculty position and I found myself suddenly on a tenure track and amongst those whom had spent their lives honing their craft as academics. I did not fit and I did not belong. As a "fish out of water," all I could do was to continue being myself. I was dealing with a foreign currency now, education, and I had better get some more if I hoped to survive. I immediately enrolled in a doctoral program while working fulltime. I was very lucky that my teaching assignment meshed with my strengths as an educator. Research wise, I wanted to make a difference, so I pursued under researched areas in education that were largely practice-based. My research informed my teaching. How I situated myself in the class was important to me. I always described myself as a facilitator in an attempt to shed the power that often accompanies being a professor. I aspired to create a democratic classroom primarily because my own learning experiences were more satisfying when that was the case. I redesigned one of the courses that I was assigned, NUTR 4444, Elements of Professional Practice. The redesign was based upon an experience I had had working with students and dietetic practitioners in the preparation of a Dietitians of Canada National Conference session. Our group had established a nonhierarchical dynamic where all views were respected. I was amazed, not only by what the students had taken on and accomplished, but with their level of professionalism and their ability to work together to communicate a difficult topic. I could envision re-creating this same success in the classroom, hence the development of NUTR 4444 workshop style with students taking the lead. I also believed it to be important for students to have a say in the topics that were covered, so put a process in place where they could brainstorm and choose the topics they wanted to learn more about. The workshops would not just be the presentation of information; they would be opportunities for students to engage and "get critical". I was thrilled at how all of this unfolded until I reviewed my course evaluations: "I want my money back – the instructor didn't teach us"; "we shouldn't have to pay for this course as we taught ourselves". While feeling quite devastated, I reflected on the situation and believed there were also many good features of the course that other students had commented on, "felt respected", "it was great that the instructor created a safe environment for us to discuss issues that had not been discussed before", or "the instructor cared and even when we got workshop feedback, it was constructive and I felt she really paid attention to our needs as students". I persisted with my approach but remain alert to student reaction and feedback. This year brought a new insight. While the classroom may be a safe space with students being able to share their feelings and reporting personal growth and deeper understandings through our work together, were we really doing the important work I had hoped in terms of critically addressing our topics? Catherine (pseudonym) in her NUTR 4444 final class reflection noted that the education system, in general, rarely exposes students to criticality. How then can they be expected to critically engage even when they arrive in a space that encourages and celebrates it? This was Catherine's experience:

> … many students had difficulty moving beyond the dominant discourses. There didn't seem to be a lot of critical analysis of issues … there was a major lack of thought given to broader factors (e.g. capitalism) that affect health, behaviours, our profession and the messages we espouse. I want to clarify here, that I am in no way blaming the individual students; rather, I place the blame on a dietetic education system that rarely exposes students to any opinions/research that challenge the positivist world view of the profession. How can we expect students to critically engage with factors affecting the profession if they are rarely given the chance, and have their opinions dismissed when they try to think this way? I have found through my time in other classes and in conversations with other students that more critical perspectives are disregarded. I had hoped that people would have engaged more these perspectives in this course since students were all so comfortable opening up to each other. (Excerpt from critical reflection paper, with permission May 1, 2018)

My assumption had been up until this point that creating a safe space would encourage the development of a more critical approach to student engagement. While students felt comfortable sharing important personal stories they were not always able to engage in critical dialogue about issues and were sometimes hesitant to share or receive beliefs or opinions that were contrary to their own.

Theory/Dialogue

I and others (Hunter 2008; Holley and Steiner 2005; Kisfalvi and Oliver 2015) sub-scribe to the importance and notion of safety and what potential it has to accomplish in the classroom; however, there are those who offer critique (Gayle et al. 2013; Redmond 2010; Barrett 2010). These tensions provide an entry point for discussion that follows about "creating a feeling of safeness", "a safe space" in an educational setting. To begin, I believe there are fundamental questions we must ask ourselves if it is possible to create such a space. What does safe space actually mean? Who are we creating the safe space for and for what purposes?

In the vignette above, the students who wanted their money back believed that I, the professor, did not teach them anything. Clearly, they wanted a highly structured teaching environment, where my expert role was to teach them what they did not know. I let them down. Did I deny them their safe space? They derived no value from developing and presenting a topic on professional practice, nor did they believe they acquired new knowledge from their peers who also delivered professional workshops. This speaks to the existence of a hierarchy of power in the classroom that not all students want to let go (Meyer and Hunt 2017; Sciull 2017). I found this somewhat disconcerting because, after all, this was the graduating year for most of these students. I wondered how they would function in the real world. hooks (1994, p. 144) observed:

> When we try to change the classroom so that there is a sense of mutual responsibility for learning, students get scared that you are now not the captain working with them, but you are after all just another crew member – and not a reliable one at that.

For me, being "just another crew member" was a signal of the respect that I had for students as young adults bringing their knowledge, experience, curiosity and questions to the classroom. All of which "I" valued. Sharing the teaching and learn-ing was a way I could divest myself of my inherent power as an academic. It was my way of inviting them into active dialogue and inquiry as a site to activate their indi-vidual and collective voices as they engaged in knowledge production. I envisioned it as a democratic space where learning and knowledge production and understand-ing could be shared. I acknowledged the power I held and continued to hold even in my attempts to redistribute it. For some of the students in the class, I had failed to deliver. The classroom that they preferred and felt safe in was the classroom in which the professor, "the expert", disseminated expert knowledge to them. This traditional model presents a challenge to achieve both student centredness and active learning (White et al. 2015). However, if students prefer lecture-style classes, it is quite plausible they are not comfortable or "safe" with the expectation that they will be asked to express an opinion or engage in discussions they feel they are ill prepared for (Meyer and Hunt 2017).

A second important contextual point to my preceding vignette relates to the actual work that can be done in a safe space. There needs to be the element of chal-lenge and not just the expression of diverse individuality (Rom 1998). The safe classroom must be more than a site where all voices are accepted. This is what frustrated Catherine; she wanted and expected tension as a site for personal challenge and subsequent growth. I did not disagree with Catherine. In my feedback to her, I acknowledged her frustration, noted the systems within the educational institution that maintain the status quo and highlighted the risks for students, in terms of further marginalization if they spoke up. I thought that for some this was the first time they may have found themselves in a space where they had a voice. However, they may still be unsure as to if and how much they wanted to disclose, even if they had a feeling of safeness.

I am reminded by the work of Cummins and Griffin (2012, p. 101) who contend that openness to voiced experience is so important to both educators and other students in the classroom. To understand and appreciate diversity in a classroom, we must first *hear* in order to respond to individual stories that, in turn, set the moral compass for any further dialogue:

> Embracing transparency, we believe that most college classrooms, including our own at times, fail to meet the needs of students of colour. Drawing from the lived experiences of our Black male student participants, they have sat in classrooms on our traditionally White campus and felt lost and excluded. As the only Black man in the class, they have had to uncomfortably ask and answer distressing questions. Arguably the most offensive to us is that they have sat in classrooms intended for learning and felt too afraid to learn. Despite the depravity in education that their disenchanting experiences reveal, we also find hope in their voiced experiences.

A safe space cannot be understood as a destination, that is, if we do x, y and z, we will get there. It is a fluid space that is constantly negotiated, and as Cummins and Griffin (2012) suggest, the safeness and meaning that any space holds can be different for everyone. Because you have a feeling of safeness in your space does not mean the person sitting beside you does. In the example above, a student of colour as a marginalized person did not feel safe. Consider other marginalized groups including lesbian, gay, bisexual and transgender (LGBT) students, as well as how students culturally identify (Holley and Steiner (2005). Sciull (2017) argues not acknowledging your audience and the diversity within the classroom can create unsafe spaces where individual identity and cultural experiences are not validated. It is difficult to feel welcome and a part of something when you are simultaneously feeling invisible or worse threatened. Until all voices are heard, how can we possibly advance our professional practice to a level where we can truly make a difference?

What do we know about safe spaces? Wilson (2013) describes a safe space as a caring space. Kisfalvi and Oliver (2015) propose that safe spaces consist of "appropriate physical aspects, trust, respect, suspension of judgement and censorship, a willingness to share and high-quality listening" (p. 713). It has been argued "that safe spaces are both 'contentious' and "'risky" … and ripe with pedagogical possibilities" (Stengel & Weems 2010, p. 506). Holley and Steiner (2005) suggest it is a space where students can openly express their authentic selves, "even if it differs dramatically from the norms set by the instructor, the profession or other student's" (p. 50). I see this as important but also a tall order for most students to achieve, as it is not easy being different and/or standing out at university. Researchers in a medium-sized tertiary institution asked students about their classroom experiences. Students reported that they were afraid and intimidated to speak up or answer questions because they did not want to be wrong (Nikolai et al. 2017). When students are active participants in learning, the classroom becomes less predictable, and potentially the students can become vulnerable depending on their engagement. For students that actively engage in discussion, they open themselves up to both critique from their instructor and fellow students (see Catherine's comments). Students may experience anxiety and fear to engage in any kind of discussion for fear of not only being wrong but also having views that are not part of dominant dietetic discourse. Gayle et al. (2013) note that as instructors, we may want students to participate in discussion; however, the more difficult the topic, the riskier it may become for them to participate. Student's efforts to be risk aversive may "stifle careful interrogation and deep learning" (Gayle et al. 2013, p. 1). In general, students want to avoid feeling criticized or ridiculed or having differing points of view (Holley and Steiner 2005). Herein lies one of the challenges of the safe space. Instructors must create space where students believe it is acceptable to make mistakes, and environments must be such that students are willing to take the risk and open themselves up to critique.

How can instructors create this kind of environment? Holley and Steiner (2005) asked students to describe the characteristics present in safe spaces. The students responded having instructors who "are knowledgeable ... share about themselves; challenge students; are laid back, flexible, or calm in the classroom; and arrange their classrooms so students can see each other" (p. 61). The notion of discussion guidelines relates to acceptable behaviour; listening and sharing were also identified as a way of supporting the safety of a classroom. Not as a mechanism to stifle critical discussion but as a safety net of sorts for when discussion was no longer productive. Instructors must engage such that they have the skills to respond (manage not rescue) to situations when "students' individualized self-expressions do not appear to be contributing to their growth ... [when] student expressions expose ideologies that impede the growth of other students ... [and] if one student's education risk is another's traumatic event" (Redmond 2010, p. 5). Redmond (2010) goes on to suggest that educators must move beyond managing dialogue to "naming why dialogue is problematic ... to maintain tension ... and to unpack ideological baggage." (pp. 9–10). This requires the vocabulary and skills to do that and some sense of why maintaining tension and unpacking words position students for more critical learning. As an educator, I too need to feel safe enough to take more risks.

Nikolai et al.' (2017) research findings resonated with me in that students preferred some learning time in small groups, interactive workshop settings, opportunities to create a place of belonging and working from within a student-focused environment. In these situations, students are gaining independence and are more self-directed in their learning (Lee and Hannafin 2016). Working from these conditions resulted in more open discussion with less fear. Students also acknowledged that they needed more practice time in class to explore learning approaches and "how to" techniques for effectively engaging in discussion (Nikolai et al. 2017). As instructors, we may take for granted that students possess these key skills and they may not.

Barrett's (2010) research presents the notion of student civility that is rooted in the civil classroom as less problematic than the metaphoric notion of safe space. Here students would be positioned as individuals within a group that would behave in a certain (civil) way. The focus is away from student comfort which may impede learning through negative experience and encourages learning though civil behaviour, active citizenship and accountability for actions (Barrett 2010).

Asking educators to create safe spaces may require a significant shift that they may be unwilling to take. Letting go of power and control, essentially relinquishing their classroom authority and their position of expert, may lead to a state of vulnerability and a sense of discomfort for them. This then becomes an "unsafe space" for the instructor. Preservation of instructor safety can, in turn, result in unsafe spaces for students by limiting student discussion, a space for students where they are denied the opportunity to develop their critical thinking and analytic skills. Kisfalvi and Oliver (2015) described this situation as regressive education. Sciull (2017) used the concept "absent audience", suggesting the lack of engagement "assumes an audience's commonality instead of recognizing its differences" (p. 238), which I have argued is important to maintain. If this is the case, instructors must question their roles in the cultivation and growth of safe spaces. Nutrition professionals and professional training programmes must look inward to determine what kind of teaching and learning space they want to model. Taking up emergent processes that will assist both faculty and students to understand their collective and individual roles in making meaningful connections in the classroom is important. This would include maintaining a reflexive approach and relinquishing the role of expert (Kisfalvi and Oliver 2015). As educators, we too must recognize that there are times that we will be vulnerable and feeling discomfort. Staying with that discomfort is critical. Through an ongoing questioning of our individual and collective places within a space, those occupying space can remain alert to the conditions required to create and maintain a safe space and manage their exposure to personal risk (Hunter 2008).

It cannot be assumed that creating a safe space will result in students approaching discussions in a more critical way; however, by practising safe space principles, I am convinced it is more likely to happen. Barrett (2010) reflects, if comfort underpins the notion of safety, is safety "conducive to (or counter to) the development of students as critical thinkers" (p. 6). My classroom was refreshing and comfortable for students. I was often told they loved Friday mornings because it was class time and they wished they had more classes like mine. I would describe them as critical thinkers, and I could see their understandings of topics growing. However, as an instructor, I would need to continuously check in and provide a level a challenge that would test both the space and students' willingness and readiness to engage within that space. I expect this intentional process would have resulted in deep critical learning that would position students to problematize in a more active way the many taken for granted actions of society and the nutrition profession. For that level of engagement, students would have had to be introduced to the notion of critical

thinking, reflection and critical dietetics as an ongoing component of their education, not just in one or two courses being offered in their senior years. Our professional programmes and processes must equip students with the foundational
competencies such as listening, reflexivity and openness in order to create and
maintain safe spaces (Kisfalvi and Oliver 2015). Key questions that I did not ask
myself, as I now reflect on the concept of safe space, that would have been useful to
me were how did I know the students had a feeling of safeness (in addition to their
obvious comfort which I could see and their ease at which they entered dialogue
about the course topics which I could hear and read), who and what are they safe for,
and what are they safe from (Stengel and Weems 2010, p. 506)?

I continue to believe that educators need to encourage the type of classroom
environment where *all* students can thrive and grow personally and professionally.
This may be the "safer space" described by Redmond (2010) or encouraging "student civility" described by Barrett (2010). It may be a yet to be defined space which
educators cocreate with learners. Whatever the situation, educators and learners
alike must be willing to ask critical questions while remaining alert to the moments
of vulnerability or "un" safety that may present themselves. Educators must be willing to wade in when moments of tension arise (Redmond 2010). Creating conditions that make risk-taking the norm should be considered part of a safe learning
environment. Understanding that "risk taking is part of academic life and intellectual growth" (Gayle et al. 2013, p. 1) can be normalized. We must not equate a
classroom devoid of tension, challenge and even distress as a safe classroom. Gayle
et al. (2013) indicated in fact the opposite could be true "participants were aware
that discomfort in a safe space was productive and lack of challenge could appear
safe, yet be dysfunctional" (p. 6). As an educator, I must continually reflect on the
differing needs and individual and collective histories of the students in the classroom and how my pedagogical choices affect the teaching environment and the
choices that students then make about engaging in critical dialogue. Safe spaces are
places where students can take risks and venture into new territory in a nonjudge-
mental way. Getting out of one's comfort zone activates personal ampowerment. I
am convinced that in order to engage in deep learning, higher-order thinking and
critical discussion, trust, a level of comfort and connection *must* be created by both
the educator and students in the class.

Section 2: Group Work Versus Team Work—Collaborative Opportunities for Development

Can you share an educational experience that resonated with you, assisted in your growth
as a student or an educator?

Student Quote

> The best group project experience that I [Jillian] ever had was very unexpected. During the semester the project was assigned, I was applying to internship and feeling the pressure to get good grades. I had been put in a group of all international students and was under a very biased impression that I would have to take on the role as the leader and editor. During the first meeting our group had, one of our members brought coffee and sweets from her country which helped us feel settled in our meeting space. Given that we were not hurried during our meeting, each member had a chance to share their ideas. We created an online document to work collaboratively on where everyone can see who added or edited what. When I logged on to upload some content, I was in disbelief by the level of participation, quality of work and feedback by all of our group members. By our last meeting we had found so many commonalities in our interests and that we had a shared (and rather twisted) sense of humour. We laughed so hard one time that tears were running down our faces and one of us fell off their chair laughing! We ended up getting an A+, but it was evident through our class and teacher feedback that the grade wasn't earned by striving to produce the typically depicted "A+" standard; it was earned through our noticeable camaraderie and supportive nature during our presentation. I acknowledge my initial ideological way of thinking that English as second language is a factor of enjoying group work. Not only do I no longer carry preconceived notions of international students, but I prefer to work with them!

Theory/Dialogue

The way we see each other is connected to the way we see ourselves. Collaborative projects are distinguishable by conceptions regarding self and other, social relations and knowledge. Valuing social inclusion and all forms of knowledge is a way to encourage praxis as an important aspect of interdisciplinary work.

Dietetics students are socialized through an "internship discourse" (Lordly and MacLellan 2012) where competitiveness transcends valuing collaboration, resulting in feelings of detachment and isolation (Atkins and Gingras 2009; Ruhl and Lordly 2017). In this competitive culture, students are pressured to stand out and get good grades as a means of receiving an internship position. This can create animosity towards group projects when students perceive one another as "not pulling their weight" and risk jeopardizing their grade. How can individuals' academic achievement, collaborative skill-building and socialization complement each other in settings where student hostility and alienation characterize the educational experience? How can pedagogy promote the kind of student success that engages larger social structural issues in a critical way? The complexities arise from opposing paradigms that are deeply embedded in the socialization of students and practitioners, telling them what is important, legitimate and reasonable (Ephross and Vassil 2005).

There is a long-standing issue in dietetics pertaining to what counts as knowledge, whereby a positivist ontology dominates the profession (Lordly 2013; Gingras et al. 2014). Not only is addressing this ideology fundamental for understanding the full scope of practice, but addressing *who* makes knowledge claims is equally imperative. The problem of students developing an internship identity in their educational experience becomes twofold when the reductionist dogma overlaps with the competitive constructs of capitalist ideology. Students are rewarded with an internship by supporting the status quo and fitting into specific professional norms. Rewarding individuals' commitments to ideological and/or value positions reinforces certain knowledge claims over others (Ladson-Billings 1995). It is here that power is comfortable and will blind individuals from other points of view and in asking critical questions about social injustices and oppression.

Dietitians' interpretive capacity to challenge objective knowledge as the conceptual currency of the profession disappears as legislative requirements increase (Lordly 2013). National systems of assessment, from regulatory bodies down to institutions, operate within a "sorting and ranking mind set" of modernity that promotes ideas for national unity (Filer 2000). The promotion and evaluation of the knowledge and skills deemed necessary for economic progress, cultural continuity and the cultivation of individual potential are reinforced by assessment criteria (Filer 2000). The scientific paradigm in which educational systems and performance standards operate under fails to include the voices of political and cultural minorities (Filer 2000). Not only are the ranking, or privileging, structures evident in student course evaluations and internship, but they veraciously underpin the research and theoretical knowledge that reasserts the value systems which inform and shape practice.

Questions about student and educator agency and contestation in and around regulation are raised if we consider the nature of dominant discourses within dietetic educational policy and the development of pedagogy. Regulatory bodies and educational systems promote student performance assessment as a means of upholding accreditation and standards of practice.

Assessment of student performance is promoted as a pedagogically desirable approach that establishes learned values. The socially co-constructed nature of this type of assessment transcends to how students interact with one another in group project work and their socialization.

While educators are under the impression that group projects mirror the "real working world", there are distinct, attention-worthy differences, which influence the overall experience of students engaging in the project as well as the quality of work and learning associated with group assignments (Brady et al. n.d.). Teamwork in the working world is reinforced by job descriptions, paid wage, potential for promotion, long-term relations with fellow colleagues and internal policies which outline consequences for poor conduct and retention of employment (Brady et al. n.d.). Given the relatively small field of dietetics and discernible policing of professionalism for internship, these guiding principles would seem applicable for dietetic students. Nonetheless, individualistic intentions appear to mask teamwork. Students' roles, responsibilities and sense of accountability differ in educational settings, and students may remain passive during team conflict or other challenges (Brady et al. n.d.).

Many students feel internally forced to think about themselves during group project work, such as by asking questions like "what will my grade be?", "when can I get this done?" and "which part should I or do I have to do?". Rather than focusing on the process of doing, students tend to focus on the project which, in turn, bypasses critical learning for professional growth. An evaluation discourse based on students' hyperawareness of performance assessment markedly applies to such circumstance.

Although the student experience written at the beginning of this section is an example of a positive scenario that supported learning and collaboration, students may be not as fortunate to have a safe space for relationship building and growth. A counterstory is apparent in Ruby's (pseudonym) reflection about a group project experience:

> Although I am an international student, I consider myself quite an extraverted person. I was very interested in the student societies on campus and participated in organizing an activity where two of the societies could go on an off-campus excursion together. During the excursion, I tried my best to meet other students but I soon became isolated by the 'clickiness' of previously bonded students. I tried very hard to make conversation with one of the students whom I had given a ride to the event, but he persisted to stare at his phone or only talk to his circle of people. I tried to brush off this negative experience. During a course in my fourth-year of the dietetics degree program, the professor assigned us groups for a major project. I was put in a group with the student who had previously alienated me. I already had mixed feelings about him but did my best to be pleasant and involved in our project. Shortly into our first group meeting, he seemed to exert the lead in the group. I was continuously interrupted and, when I did have the chance to speak, he would dismiss my ideas. I mustered up the courage to speak one-on-one with him. I told him how I felt left out and disrespected, and that perhaps it was because we never had a chance to connect. He unapologetically agreed to be more responsive in including me in the group. It never ended up happening and I carry a negative memory about the project and group members. (Excerpt from email dialogue, with permission, May 2, 2018)

It is clear in this scenario that the experiences, biases and power relations of particular cultural groups failed to incorporate culturally and socially diverse perspectives. The embedded assumptions about knowledge and individual student achievement, inscribed in the assessment process, may have contributed to the hierarchical relations exercised by the group members.

Addressing student achievement while helping students accept and affirm their cultural identity is necessary to gain an appreciation for other forms of knowledge and, thus, develop critical perspectives. Educators working under a critical pedagogy understand the merit of assigning group projects in which students learn to be open to diversity and socially tolerant and develop interpersonal skills (Romero 1998). Without critical pedagogy, students (as future practitioners) will devalue historical and cultural narratives, while not seeking alternative emancipatory discourse within education (Stromquist 1998). Ladson-Billings (1995) used the term "culturally relevant pedagogy" to describe a theoretical model that posits effective pedagogical practice as challenging the inequities perpetuated by schools and institutions. Making small changes in everyday participation structures may be one of the means to which more culturally responsive pedagogy can be developed. One of the means in which educators could achieve this is by incorporating small group discussions and mini in-class assignments that require collaborative skill-building and dialogue for participation marks. This would give students the opportunity to interact with many of their peers while not bearing the weight and stress of being heavily evaluated on a major group project.

Integrating diverse academic and social activities into a meaningful whole is necessary for experiential learning and growth (Zhao and Kuh 2014). What might happen to learning and practice if dietetic students strived to meet their competency statement in a direct manner, like a checklist? While fulfilling competency statements can accomplish and delineate specific skills, it can often overlook critical and reflexive learning for practice. For example, when given the task of assessing a specific population's health and increasing their nutritional status, a dietetic student might design an educational tool for the target group. With the task of finishing the assignment, the student may often jump to conclusions about the needs and implementation of their tool. Rather than focusing on the actual tool and outcome, students need to focus on making connections with the target group at hand in order to grasp a full understanding of the world in which they live and see through. This requires collaborative conversations, valuing all forms of knowledge and reflexively thinking about the power structures and discursive practices influencing one another's quality of life. By learning to approach discussion in this way, we are setting ourselves up to be able to collaboratively work with others towards optimal care and wellness. This same principle of learning applies to teamwork among peers in higher education. Making connections and building authentic relationships with peers require an equal distribution of power and a willingness to embrace vulnerability. All team members must actively listen and participate and assist in the creation of a comfortable environment that enables members to do so. Harnessing the unique skillsets and characteristics of individuals, teaching one another, relieving possible feelings of peer alienation and valuing the academic success of others are vital learning experiences that should be cherished when partaking in group projects.

However obviously stated, group project work cannot be viewed individualistically. Knowledge emerges in dialectical relationships (Ladson-Billings 1995). Rather than the voice of one individual, meaning and values are cultivated through dialogue and connections between and among individuals. The terms team and group are often used interchangeably; however, there is a remarkable difference between the two (Brady et al. n.d.). A team is a much more powerful connection than a group as it entails working together with a great level of commitment and mutual respect towards one another, beyond simply coming together for a common purpose (Brady et al. n.d.). As Brady et al. (n.d.) wrote, "All teams are groups, but not all groups are teams".

Reflecting on the examples of student experiences reveals the diffusion of individualism from regulation to the educational system to student camaraderie. The highly contested debate of how educational systems inscribe dominate values, mainly through the assessment process, must continue to be challenged. Professional narratives have real-life consequences (Aphramor 2018). The changing and often conflicting priorities for educational policy require its own evaluation of the power and knowledge it generates. Discovering the small differences in social relations makes a big difference in the interactional ways in which students engage with the content of curriculum and their developing identities. *Real* teamwork prepares students and practitioners for confronting inequitable and undemocratic social structures. Students, educators and practitioners must give full consideration to new and diverse perspectives in order to build an effective and caring workforce. They need to be receptive and responsive to different ways of talking, acting and seeing the world. For students, dismantling the rogue of group work under individualistic intentions is one starting block of opening up new streams of knowledge. For educators and practitioners, a shift in pedagogical practice and approaches for care that focus on the complex sociocultural settings of learners and clients is warranted. Lastly, a trauma-informed approach deserves the immediate attention of all professionals in order to challenge the scientific paradigms that perpetuate individualism (Aphramor 2018); for to learn the narratives of others is to learn of the self (Gingras 2008).

Section 3: Creating a Non-judging Workforce

Can you share an educational experience that resonated with you, assisted in your growth as a student or an educator?

Teacher Quote

I [Elin] was leading a seminar with a small group of students. The seminar focused at a patient case describing a person with a long experience of unemployment and depressive-like symptoms. The person had, during recent years, gained weight as food and eating had a comforting role in his life. The students' task during the seminar was to formulate a suitable description of his nutrition problem that could be documented in his patient record. One of the students suggested using the phrase, "involuntary weight gain", and others agreed. Another student however opposed, stating "I believe there is no involuntary weight gain. Everybody knows that if you eat more than you need, you will gain weight. I'm sure this patient also knew that. Thus, I agree the problem is weight gain, but I would rather call it voluntary". Several of the other students reacted to this statement, which they found judgemental. They argued that knowledge is not enough to change people's behaviour, as our eating habits and other health-related behaviour are affected by cultural or social aspects rather than merely our knowledge level. The seminar turned into a discussion about individuals' health-related responsibility in society, our approaches as dietetic and nutrition professionals and the role of empathy and compassion in the dietetic and nutrition profession.

Theory/Dialogue

Society today is dominated by an individualist health discourse, implying assumptions such that an individual's health behaviour is mainly driven by himself or herself (Korp 2010; Holm 2015). This discourse does not take into account the complex context consisting of sociopolitical, cultural and environmental norms and conventions and financial boundaries. The individualist discourse incorporates an assumption that human behaviours depend on the individual's own thinking and deliberation, rather than from bodily signals or social conventions. Thus, according to this perspective, information is enough to change a person's health behaviour. However, research has shown that information is not enough and that health behaviour is largely affected by social and cultural aspects, rather than individual driving forces (Halkier and Jensen 2011; Holm 2015). Furthermore, this individualist discourse is tightly connected to the stigmatization of "unhealthy" lifestyles, as it incorporates the basic assumption that individuals are responsible for their own choices and, therefore, blamed when they fail to maintain health (the dominant discourse) (Korp 2010).

The individualist and cognitivist health discourse (Howarth et al. 2004; Korp 2010) that is present in all parts of society today creates the need for a dialogue between students and teachers about the assumptions inherent within. Often, students have their own stories to share regarding food-related problems or experiences from health-care settings. In a systematic review study, it was found that students' empathy levels often decline during medical education and training (Neumann et al. 2011). The suggested reasons for this decline were that encountering morbidity and mortality might increase the students' own feelings of vulnerability. As a reaction to this, the students protected themselves by dehumanizing the patient.

The concept of empathy can be understood and practised on different levels. According to psychologist Singer and Klimecki (2014), the highest level of empathy, called compassion, is characterized by a feeling of concern for another person's suffering and connected to the motivation to help. Furthermore, it is associated with a practical approach of applying this feeling of empathy into action. The lower degrees of empathy, in contrast, are more self-related and connected to negative feelings like stress and burnout.

How can we all participate in the creation of an empathetic, compassionate and non-judging dietetic workforce? How can we, during our education, train ourselves to see beyond the individualist discourse and, instead, develop an understanding for the complex web of societal, cultural and physiological aspects that affect human behaviour?

Literature in nursing and medical training suggest several approaches for educating and training students in empathy, often involving nontraditional teaching approaches such as role-playing and art-based learning. Some of this literature is described below.

Cunico et al. (2012) developed an empathy training course for nursing students, including movie frames followed by a guided examination of the situation concerning the relationship between nurse and patient/family. Other parts of the course included individual and pair exercises on communication skills, role-playing and discussions. Evaluating the training course with a questionnaire, the authors could show that these approaches really had an effect on the nursing students' empathy levels.

Storytelling as a teaching approach in health care has been highlighted by McAllister et al. (2009), emphasizing that narratives contribute to an increased understanding of the real feeling of an experience, rather than the external perspectives that often characterize education in health-care professions. Brady and Gingras (2012) discussed the narrative teaching approach more specifically related to dietetic education and training. It was concluded that storytelling has the potential to create greater empathy and connection between educators and students, practitioners and their patients/clients. Davidhizar and Lonser (2003) suggested three main ways in which storytelling can enrich nursing education: (1) use of stories that role model different kinds of nursing interventions and illustrate concepts; (2) use of case studies, scenarios and vignettes for analysis; and (3) use of reflective analysis.

Including narrative literature has also been highlighted as a way of increasing students' empathy and understanding for patients' situations. At the University of Southern Mississippi, narrative non-fiction literature (*The Immortal Life of Henrietta Lacks* by Rebecca Skloot) was incorporated into a medical nutrition course (Rupp and Huye 2017). Regular readings and book club meetings resulted in a rich discussion about empathy in the health-care field, and students concluded that this teaching approach was eye opening, provided new perspectives and helped them to become more empathetic health-care professionals (Rupp and Huye 2017). Perkin and Rodriguez (2013) argued for the inclusion of nontraditional literature in dietetic education, as this can help students to better understand the impact of a disease or disorder in a person's life. They suggested that dietetic education should include titles like *Being Ana: A Memoir of Anorexia Nervosa*, by Shani Raviv, or *The Last of the Husbandmen: A Novel of Farming Life* by Gene Logsdon.

Empathy and adherence to ethical approaches are described as parts of a professional approach. In education and training of health-care professionals, "professionalism" is often used as an umbrella concept, containing specialist knowledge and skills and reflective practice (Brody and Doukas 2014; Nortje 2017). Grace and Trede (2013, p. 803) suggested five main strategies for developing a strong sense of professionalism among dietetic students:

1. Students look to their lecturers and clinical educators as role models of professionalism.
2. There is a need for reflective spaces to learn and make sense of professionalism in the workplace and at university (especially after workplace experiences) to critically reflect and make meaning of them.
3. Lecturers need to create capacity in students to question and discuss professionalism from philosophical perspectives and as active participants.
4. Students learn from talking about professionalism.

5. Discussions about professionalism need to include contemporary social and cultural issues as they relate to professional practice.

Going back to the scenario described above, the patient case discussion caused reactions among the students in the seminar group. There are several aspects that I believe affected their reactions and our discussion, among which the most important might be the way we see health – as depending mainly on the individuals themselves or being a result of societal and cultural aspects such as social conventions or financial constraints. Some students reacted rather strongly on what they perceived as a judging statement, blaming an individual for problems that to them seemed to be caused by aspects out of his control, that is, unemployment and depression. On the other hand, some students were provoked by the statement that the patient himself should not be seen as responsible for his own situation. It is not a coincidence that this discussion was raised regarding a weight-focused patient case. The stigmatization of nonnormative body size and the blaming of individuals for "unhealthy" lifestyles have been described and discussed by several scholars, as a factor that contributes to poor quality of life among people who do not live up to the societal norm regarding body size and shape (Brandheim 2017; Daníelsdóttir et al. 2010; Warschburger 2005). Scholars have suggested an alternative health framework focusing on health and wellbeing rather than weight results, describing compassion and connection as important aspects when supporting patients (Aphramor 2005; Brady et al. 2013). This framework is a valuable resource in discussions about dietitians' responsibilities in the development of a person-centred care.

In society today, people are to a great extent seen as responsible for their own health and expected to choose a healthy lifestyle based on a rational choice. An unhealthy lifestyle is seen as a conscious choice, which the individual can be blamed for, even though we know that our behaviour and approach towards food and eating are affected by cultural and societal aspects. The dietetic professional needs a critical approach towards this dominating discourse to be able to fully understand the patient and his or her situation, which in turn is needed to be able to help the patient and to provide a truly person-centred nutrition care. This needs to start during dietetic and nutrition education. Although empathy and compassion should be considered as essential competencies among dietetic professionals, these aspects seem to have been excluded to a great extent from the nutrition and dietetics curriculum. Definitely, an important goal to strive for is the inclusion of these aspects in the curriculum and other steering documents. While working on that process, the inclusion of creative and arts-based teaching methods within our professional education and training programmes would be a good start (Lordly 2014; Fox et al. 2017).

This inclusion would contribute to the development of a future dietetic workforce that would appreciate approaching practice with curiosity and understanding for each individual patient and his or her situation.

Section 4: The Critical Classroom

Our theme, awakening the possibilities, and our subsections highlight there is still work to be done in terms of cocreating a critically informed nutrition and dietetics professional training and education practice. Currently, elements of our profession rely heavily on a positivist informed paradigm to (re)produce a practice that is thought to more favourably align itself with dominant medical thinking (Gingras et al. 2014). Critical practitioners understand the confines of such a position. They strive to broaden and deepen professional perspectives in order for students to develop more informed, reflexive and sustainable practices that will position them to address current and future issues in authentic and meaningful ways. As such, we reached out to these practitioners and asked them what a critical classroom would look like. In addressing these questions, we would also like you to reflect on and consider an observation that was offered:

> I used to think getting rid of theatre style, sitting in circles, and/or sharing teaching with students could help equalize power, but now I think it just places it in different forms, moving position power/surveillance power to disciplinary power/self-surveillance.

In what ways might power exert itself in the classroom and how might you respond? Why might it be important to acknowledge and respond to such relations?

What follows are selected practitioner responses for discussion:

> The classroom would be colourful … writing and arts-based modes of teaching/learning displayed on the walls.

> There would be "space" – I see the classroom as existing outside the physical walls; it would work on bringing experience and context into learning in order to keep complexity/ambiguity of health/humanity alive.

> There would be a sense of belonging in the classroom. The space would feel alive, a risky place to enter that was nevertheless, despite some trepidation, strangely compelling.

> It would be a mixture of quiet and loud – time for self-reflection/internal thought and time for discussions.

> It would be a place where vulnerability is encouraged – the educator would be modelling critical humility (a sense of confidence amidst partiality/openness that interpretations are wrong/mistakes are going to be made) and courageous vulnerability (bringing self-doubts, self-questioning, self-forgiveness into the classroom).

> It would be critically nurturing – where relationships were built with the educator, students feel cared for yet pushed.
>
> It would look like a variety of activities (individual reflection, conversations, reading, art – storytelling, poetry, metaphors, images – and experiential activities (role plays, simulations, body movement to learn/represent concepts/definitions) were happening.

> Bodies, subjectivities, emotions, stories would be brought into reflections/discussions.

It would be a space where both objectivity and subjectivity would be valued; discussing the value of integrating reason/intuition and objectivity/subjectivity.

Tolerance for uncertainty and ambiguity would be promoted.

Intersectionality would be examined/explored and privilege would be explicitly named, discovering its impacts/reinforcement of inequity.

Discussions would consider what was missing in a curious versus an overly critical way. In particular missing voices and histories.
    A variety of modes of knowing and "types" of evidence would be introduced. There would be active discussion around what all types of knowing and evidence can and cannot do.

The politics of knowledge and whose knowledge "counts" and why would be examined.

In dietetics the three traditional roles for RDs; clinical, community/population health and food service/management would be problematized.
    Learning spaces would incorporate qualities like kindness, empathy and compassion as the fundamental underpinning to competent, safe and ethical practice as is technical proficiency.

As you consider these responses, we would like you to consider how the ideas, if you have not yet experienced them in your learning environments, would lead to a different kind of professional knowing? How could these ideas be operationalized in your classrooms and practice? Returning to your mind map at the beginning of this chapter, reflect on your educational experiences and how they relate to the content of this chapter.
    How might the possibilities inherent in the above practices awaken your critical self?

Acknowledgements We would like to thank the critical dietetics and nutrition practitioners who offered their passionate insights and suggestions for creating critical classrooms.

Assignments

1. Think about a class you took in which you felt a sense of safeness. What was the educator doing or not doing? What were the students doing or not doing? What was it about the physical space that contributed or took away from your sense of safeness? Using strips of paper provided by your instructor, print words or short phases that describe the aspects of contributors to feelings of safeness in black marker – one idea per strip. Simultaneously, using a red marker, print words or short phases that describe the detractors of creating a safe space or feelings of safeness in the classroom.
    Break into small groups (4–5 students), and discuss your individual results with your group. What did you notice?

Within your small groups, reflect on the following questions:

- What are some ideas that were presented by your group members that you had not previously considered in your understanding of safe space?
- How important is a safe space to be able to engage in deep, critical learning or learning that pushes you beyond your current understandings?
- How does your understanding of safe space influence your willingness to raise controversial thoughts or ideas that are not part of the dominant professional discourse?
- Safe spaces can sometimes lead to spaces of vulnerability for both the person sharing and the person(s) actively receiving or listening. Are these learning spaces? In what ways?

Transfer all of the strips of paper to the two large boards provided by the educator. One board will display the contributor descriptors and the other the detractor descriptors. Take a few moments to reflect on what you see. Within the large group, discuss the following:

- What are your most meaningful insights/learnings emerging from the safe spaces that your group and the large group were able to describe?
- What are your thoughts regarding "safe space"?
- Whom is being kept safe from what? What is gained or lost through creating a safe space?
- What possibilities do the concept of safe space offer you as you develop your skills in critical nutrition and dietetics?

2. Critical Consciousness Exercise

The process of critical consciousness includes three phases: (1) identifying the ideologies and assumptions that underlie our thoughts and actions; (2) scrutinizing the accuracy and validity of these in terms of how they connect to, or are discrepant with, our experience of reality; and (3) reconstructing these assumptions to make them more inclusive and integrative (Norris 2014). Recognition and analysis of ideological assumptions are central to the process of critical reflection (Norris 2014). Ideologies can be defined as the enduring sense that a person has of ones' identity, such as gender, sexual orientation, ethnicity and class (Lee et al. 2007), and comprises of those taken for granted ideas, commonsense beliefs and self-evident "rules" that inform our thoughts and actions (Norris 2014).

Reflect on the narrative in Section 3 about the students who were influenced in their attitudes and assumptions towards body weight. Was there a time in which you felt ideological towards someone or a group or a time in which you yourself felt stigmatized? If you feel comfortable, share your story to your small group. Describe the details of the situations, such as the time, place and people (while keeping the names of the people involved anonymous) and the reason(s) why that event resonates with you. What similarities or differences were discovered between the stories shared within your group? What core ideologies and discursive practices do you think were present in these situations and inform both you and your group members' selection of these critical incidents? What are the consequences of these assumptions? As a group, jot down any thoughts, words or phrases on paper of the connecting elements and relationships in which these actions ensue. How can we as dietetic and nutrition professionals resist or change these attitudes and actions which perpetuate judgement and stigma?

3. In what ways might the concepts and propositions from critical dietetics and nutrition contribute to a more inclusive and authentic education? Did the elements of critical practice addressed in this chapter resonate with you? Moving forward, what practices and processes will you engage in that you believe will result in a more critical practice?

Definition of Keywords and Terms

Ampowerment	Refers to a meaningful sense of one's power-from-within (Aphramor 2016). The term ampowerment is coined by Lucy Aphramor. As Aphramor explains, "Lifestyle change falls under the rubric of ampowerment, which relates to self-care. Ampowerment fosters empowerment through links with a critical awareness of power-over, and increased capacity to engage in and influence power-with relationships. Empowerment is a process that involves systemic social change, with action preceded by collective consciousness raising. It does not stop at self-esteem. It is not about compliance or co-ercion" (Aphramor 2016).
Discourse	"A series of representations, practices, and performances through which meanings are produced, connected into networks, and legitimized. Discourses are heterogeneous, regulated, embedded, situated, and performative" (Gingras 2009, p. 238).
Ideology	Refers, traditionally, to the relatively stable and enduring sense that a person has of ones' identity, such as gender, sexual orientation, ethnicity and class (Lee et al. 2007).
Individualism	Refers to the conception of an individual being the essential proprietor of one's own capacities, owing nothing to society for them (Macpherson 1962).
Narrative	A story or account of events, interactions and experiences that are selectively recalled, arranged and interpreted by a person, family or community. Narratives serve to organize and give meaning to the story teller(s) (Lee et al. 2007).
Ontology	Refers to the branch of philosophy that deals with being (Lee et al. 2007).
Other	Refers to the attempt to form a personal or group identity and where comparison of ourselves to others creates an understanding of ourselves as separate and different from others. The process of comparison can establish identity but can also create a sense of

superiority and an objectification of those who are "different" (Lee et al. 2007).

Praxis   Refers to the unity of theory and practice (Lee et al. 2007).

Reflexivity   Understood to be different from reflection in that reflection can involve an actor examining an object, whereas reflexivity is an internal conversation where an embodied actor in a social context bends their thoughts back on themselves (Vink et al. 2017).

How This Chapter Addresses the Critical Dietetics Framework

When we, as authors, came together to discuss our subsections, we were struck, but the obvious interconnections were present. Daphne reflected on the importance of creating the conditions for a space where students and professors could engage in conversations that were insightful, respectful, critical and real, spaces where all class members could add their voices to the dialogue and that there could be a deep understanding and unpacking of moments of tension and (dis)ease. Jillian called for the bringing together of individuals to work collaboratively as teams. She highlighted the dominant structures in place that are often challenges to achieving inclusive learning and teamwork. How we as individuals set ourselves up for collaborative work requires a breaking down of stereotypes and bias in order to connect and function in meaningful ways. If shared meaning and values are to be fostered, the cocreation of a space in which that can happen is imperative. Elin also highlights the troubling consequences of a focus on the individual. She argues for the advancement of empathetic, compassionate and non-judging professionals. These characteristics are fostered in teams and in spaces where individuals connect and develop a greater awareness and understanding of themselves and each other.

References

Aphramor L (2005) Is a weight-centred health framework salutogenic? Some thoughts on unhinging certain dietary ideologies. Soc Theory Health 3(4):315–340. Accessed 8 May 2018 from SpringerLink, ISSN; 1477-822X

Aphramor L (2016) Well now: radical dietitian, glossary. http://lucyaphramor.com/dietitian/glossary/. Accessed 20 May 2018

Aphramor L (2018) Why we need to talk about trauma in public health nutrition. Public Health 133(April):37–40. www.NHDmag.com

Atkins J, Gingras J (2009) Coming and going: dietetic students' experience of their education. Can J Diet Pract Res 70:181–186. Accessed 15 Jan 2018 Dietitians of Canada. https://doi.org/10.3148/70.4.2009.181

Barrett BJ (2010) Is "safety" dangerous? A critical examination of the classroom as safe space. Can J Scholarsh Teach Learn 1(1):Article 9. https://doi.org/10.5206/cjsotl-rcacea.2010.1.9. Accessed 1 Feb 2018

Brady J, Gingras J (2012) Dietetics students' experiences and perspectives of storytelling to enhance food and nutrition practice. Transform Dialogues Teach Learn J 6(1):1–12. https://www.kpu.ca/sites/default/files/Teaching%20and%20Learning/TD.6.1.11_Brady%26Gingras_Stories_in_Food%26Nutrition.pdf. Accessed 15 Jan 2018

Brady J, Gingras J, Aphramor L (2013) Theorizing health at every size as a relational–cultural endeavour. Crit Public Health 23(3):345–355. Accessed 2 Mar 2018 from Taylor & Francis Online. https://doi.org/10.1080/09581596.2013.797565

Brady J, Farrell A, Fleming L, Liu A, Smith D, Dejonge L (n.d.) SPARC guide: supporting partnerships to advance results of collaboration. Ryerson University, pp 1–26, https://www.ryerson.ca/castl/resources/SPARC_Guide/SPARC_Guide1_0.pdf. Accessed 5 Jan 2018

Brandheim S (2017) A systemic stigmatization of fat people. PhD, Karlstads University Studies, Sweden

Brody H, Doukas D (2014) Professionalism: a framework to guide medical education. Med Educ 48(10):980–987. Accessed 4 Jan 2018 from Wiley Online Library. https://doi.org/10.1111/medu.12520

Cummins MW, Griffin RA (2012) Critical race theory and critical communication pedagogy: articulating pedagogy as an act of love from black male perspectives. Liminalities J Perform Stud 8(5):85–106. Accessed 4 Jan 2018, ISSN; 12-2935

Cunico L, Sartori R, Marognolli O, Meneghini AM (2012) Developing empathy in nursing students: a cohort longitudinal study. J Clin Nurs 21(13–14):2016–2025. Accessed 15 February 2018 from Wiley Online Library. https://doi.org/10.1111/j.1365-2702.2012.04105.x

Daníelsdóttir S, O'brien KS, Ciao A (2010) Anti-fat prejudice reduction: a review of published studies. Obes Facts 3(1):47–58. https://doi.org/10.1159/000277067. Accessed 1 Feb 2018

Davidhizar R, Lonser G (2003) Storytelling as a teaching technique. Nurse Educ 28(5):217–221. Accessed 1 Feb 2018 from The National Center for Biotechnology Information (NCBI), PMID: 14506353

Ephross PH, Vassil TV (2005) Groups that work: structure and process, 2nd edn. Columbia University Press, New York

Filer A (2000) Assessment: social practice and social product. Routledge, London

Fox A, Gillis D, Anderson B, Lordly D (2017) Stronger together: use of storytelling at a dietetics conference to promote professional collaboration. Can J Diet Pract Res 78(1):32–36. Accessed 15 Jan 2018 from Dietitians of Canada. https://doi.org/10.3148/cjdpr-2016-027

Gayle BM, Cortez D, Preiss RW (2013) Safe spaces, difficult dialogues, and critical thinking. Int J Scholarsh Teach Learn 7(2):1–8, Article 5. https://doi.org/10.20429/ijsotl.2013.070205. Accessed 4 Mar 2018

Gingras J (2008) The vulnerable learner: moving from middle to margin in dietetic education. Transform Dialogues Teach Learn J 1(3):1–5. https://www.kpu.ca/sites/default/files/Teaching%20and%20Learning/TD.1.3_Gingras_Vulnerable_Learner.pdf. Accessed 8 Jan 2018

Gingras J (2009) Longing for recognition: The joys, complexities, and contradictions of practicing dietetics. MPG Biddles Ltd. King's Lynn, Norfolk

Gingras J, Asada Y, Fox A, Coveney J, Berenbaum S, Aphramor L (2014) Critical dietetics: a discussion paper. J Crit Diet 2(1):2–12. Accessed 15 Dec 2017 from ResearchGate, ISSN; 1923-1237

Grace S, Trede F (2013) Developing professionalism in physiotherapy and dietetics students in professional entry courses. Stud High Educ 38(6):793–806. Accessed 4 Mar 2018 from Taylor & Francis Online. https://doi.org/10.1080/03075079.2011.603410

Halkier B, Jensen I (2011) Doing 'healthier' food in everyday life? A qualitative study of how Pakistani Danes handle nutritional communication. Crit Public Health 21(4):471–483. Accessed 20 Jan 2018 from Taylor & Francis Online. https://doi.org/10.1080/09581596.2011.594873

Holley LC, Steiner S (2005) Safe space: student perspectives on classroom environment. J Soc Work Educ 41(1):49–64. Accessed 12 Mar 2018 from Elsevier, ISSN; 1043-7797

Holm L (2015) Explaining consumer choice: a critique of the theory of planned behaviour. In: The consumer in society. Abstrakt forlag, Oslo, pp 123–148. Accessed 4 Feb 2018

hooks b (1994) Teaching to transgress: education as the practice of freedom. Routledge, New York

Howarth C, Foster J, Dorrer N (2004) Exploring the potential of the theory of social representations in community-based health research – and vice versa? J Health Psychol 9(2):229–243. Accessed 1 Feb 2018 from SAGE Journals. https://doi.org/10.1177/1359105304040889

Hunter MA (2008) Cultivating the art of safe space. Res Drama Educ 13(1):5–21. Accessed 5 Feb 2018 from Taylor & Francis Online. https://doi.org/10.1080/13569780701825195

Kisfalvi V, Oliver D (2015) Creating and maintaining a safe space in experiential learning. J Manag Educ 39(6):713–740. Accessed 15 Mar 2018 from SAGE Journals. https://doi.org/10.1177/1052562915574724

Korp P (2010) Problems of the healthy lifestyle discourse. Sociol Compass 4(9):800–810. Accessed 20 Jan 2018 from Wiley Online Library. https://doi.org/10.1111/j.1751-9020.2010.00313.x

Ladson-Billings G (1995) Toward a theory of culturally relevant pedagogy. Am Educ Res J 32(3):465–491. Accessed 9 Jan 2018 from JSTOR. https://doi.org/10.2307/1163320

Lee E, Hannafin MJ (2016) A design framework for enhancing engagement in student-centered learning: own it, learn it, and share it. Educ Technol Res Dev 64:707–734. Accessed 4 Jan 2018 from ERIC, ISSN; ISSN-1042-1629

Lee B, Sammon S, Dumbrill GC (2007) Glossary of terms for anti oppressive policy & practice. Common Act Press, Mississauga

Lordly D (2013) Dietetics prior learning assessment: a Canadian study about what counts as dietetic knowledge. DEd, University of South Australia

Lordly D (2014) Crafting meaning: arts-informed dietetics education. Can J Diet Pract Res 75(2):89–94. Accessed 2 Feb 2018 from Dietitians of Canada. https://doi.org/10.3148/75.2.2014.89

Lordly D, MacLellan D (2012) Dietetic students' identity and professional socialization. Can J Diet Prac Res 73:7–13. Accessed 8 Jan 2018 from Dietitians of Canada. https://doi.org/10.3148/73.1.2012.7

Macpherson CB (1962) The political theory of possessive individualism: Hobbes to Locke. Clarendon Press, Oxford

McAllister M, John T, Gray M, Williams L, Barnes M, Allan J, Rowe J (2009) Adopting narrative pedagogy to improve the student learning experience in a regional Australian university. Contemp Nurse 32(1–2):156–165. Accessed 4 Mar 2018 from The National Center for Biotechnology Information (NCBI), PMID: 19697986

Meyer KR, Hunt SK (2017) The lost art of lecturing: cultivating student listening and Notetaking. Commun Educ 66(2):239–241. Accessed 15 Jan 2018 from Taylor & Francis Online. https://doi.org/10.1080/03634523.2016.1275719

Neumann M, Edelhäuser F, Tauschel D, Fischer MR, Wirtz M, Woopen C, Haramati A, Scheffer C (2011) Empathy decline and its reasons: a systematic review of studies with medical students and residents. Acad Med 86(8):996–1009. Accessed 1 Feb 2018 from Wolters Kluwer. https://doi.org/10.1097/ACM.0b013e318221e615

Nikolai J, Silva P, Walters S (2017) Student and lecturer perspectives informing an academic support strategy to assist students in a medium-sized tertiary institution. ATLAANZ J 2(1):1–18. Accessed 2 Feb 2018 from Research Gate. https://doi.org/10.26473/atlaanz.2017.2.1/001

Norris D (2014) Critical Theories in Family Studies and Gerontology (GFSG 6613) Assignments. Winter 2014 Semester Course Syllabus. Mount Saint Vincent University, Nova Scotia

Nortje N (2017) Attributes contributing to the development of professionalism as described by dietetics students. S Afr J Clin Nutr 30(1):21–23. Accessed 15 Mar 2018 from Taylor & Francis Online. https://doi.org/10.1080/16070658.2016.1225367

Perkin JE, Rodriguez JC (2013) More lit can fit: using nontraditional literature in dietetics education to enhance cultural competence, cultural literacy, and critical thinking. J Acad Nutr Diet 113(6):758. Accessed 2 Feb 2018 from ScienceDirect. https://doi.org/10.1016/j.jand.2013.01.028

Redmond M (2010) Safe space oddity: revisiting critical pedagogy. J Teach Soc Work 30(1):1–14. Accessed 5 Mar 2018 from Taylor & Francis Online. https://doi.org/10.1080/08841230903249729

Rom RB (1998) 'Safe spaces': reflections on an educational metaphor. J Curric Stud 30(4):397–408. Accessed 20 Mar 2018. https://doi.org/10.20429/ijsotl.2013.070205

Romero MMRR (1998) Educational change and discourse communities: representing change in postmodern times. Curric Stud 6(1):47–71. Accessed 8 Jan 2018 from Taylor & Francis Online. https://doi.org/10.1080/14681369800200026

Ruhl J, Lordly D (2017) The nature of competition in dietetics education: a narrative review. Can J Diet Prac Res 78:129–136. Accessed 17 Jan 2018 from Dietitians of Canada. https://doi.org/10.3148/cjdpr-2017-004

Rupp R, Huye H (2017) Using humanities content in a medical nutrition therapy course to enhance empathy in senior nutrition students. J Acad Nutr Diet 117(9):A38. Accessed 15 Jan 2018 from ScienceDirect. https://doi.org/10.1016/j.jand.2017.06.300

Sciull NJ (2017) The lecture's absent audience. Commun Educ 66(2):236–255. Accessed 2 Feb 2018 from Taylor & Francis Online. https://doi.org/10.1080/03634523.2016.1275722

Singer T, Klimecki OM (2014) Empathy and compassion. Curr Biol 24(18):R875–R878. Accessed 20 Jan 2018 from ScienceDirect. https://doi.org/10.1016/j.cub.2014.06.054

Stengel B, Weems L (2010) Questioning safe space: an introduction. Stud Philos Educ 29(6):505–507. Accessed 2 Feb 2018 from PhilPapers. https://doi.org/10.1007/s11217-010-9205-8

Stromquist, NP (1998, November 4) The challenges of emancipation in higher education. Paper presented as part of a keynote speech, ASHE International Pre-conference, Miami, pp 1–12

Vink J, Wetter-Edman K, Aguirre M (2017) Designing for aesthetic disruption: Altering mental models in social systems through designerly practices. Des J 20(Sup 1):S2168–S2177. Accessed 5 July 2018 from Taylor & Francis Online. https://doi.org/10.1080/14606925.2017.1352733

Warschburger P (2005) The unhappy obese child. Int J Obes 29(S2):S127. Accessed 10 Feb 2018 from Taylor & Francis Online, ISSN; 0307-0565

White PJ, Larson I, Styles K, Yuriev E, Evans DR, Rangachari PK, Short JL, Exintaris B, Malone DT, Davie B, Eise N, McNamara K, Naidu S (2015) Adopting an active learning approach to teaching in a research-intensive higher education context transformed staff teaching attitudes and Behaviours. High Educ Res Dev 35(3):619–633. Accessed 15 Jan 2018 from Nature, ISSN; 0729-4360

Wilson S (2013) Caring leadership applied in the classroom to embrace the needs of students. J Coll Learn 10(1):23–28. Accessed 10 Mar 2018 from ERIC, ISSN; ISSN-1544-0389

Zhao CM, Kuh GD (2014) Adding value: learning communities and student engagement. Res High Educ 45(2):115–138. Accessed 14 Dec 2017 from Springer Link, ISSN; 0361-0365

Chapter 5
Critical Perspectives in Clinical Nutrition Practice

Catherine Morley

Aim of Chapter and Learning Outcomes

The aim of this chapter is to familiarize readers with forms of power including power over and being powered over, to outline how these may be present in clinical nutrition practice, and to suggest possible actions to disrupt forms of power that negatively affect client-centeredness.

At the end of this chapter, the readers will be able to:

Describe the meanings of *power over* and *being powered over.*
Identify and describe at least eight forms of power.
Describe how forms of power relate to clinical nutrition practice and provide examples.
Describe how client-centeredness relates to forms of power in clinical nutrition practice.
Describe approaches at least two ways to disrupt forms of power.

Summary

Providing nutritional care in clinical settings is inherently complex and calls upon the practitioner to recognize and balance multiple forms of power and competing demands and interests. These include relationships with patients/clients/residents and their family/friends, coworkers, and managers/senior administrators who all have expectations of what nutritional care should entail and the role of the dietitian. This chapter contains ideas on approaching practice in clinical settings to optimize

C. Morley (✉)
Acadia University, Wolfville, NS, Canada
e-mail: catherine.morley@acadiau.ca

© Springer Nature Switzerland AG 2019
J. Coveney, S. Booth (eds.), *Critical Dietetics and Critical Nutrition Studies,*
Food Policy, https://doi.org/10.1007/978-3-030-03113-8_5

client-centered nutritional care recognizing that biological needs are one of many considerations. The reader is invited to consider how such a shift in focus might (or could, or perhaps ought to) disrupt forms of power.

Declaration of Intent

In this chapter, I outline and explore the dominant forms of power (*power over* and *powered over*) in settings where clinical nutrition is practiced (typically hospitals, clinics, residential care) and consider the value of recognizing and addressing forms of power to optimize nutritional care and quality of work life for clinical dietitians. I advocate a post-oppositional perspective (*"transformative modes of engagement that move through oppositional approaches to embrace interconnectivity as a framework for identity formation, theorizing, social change, and the possibility of planetary citizenship"* (Keating 2013)). This invites those holding power to recognize their privilege and to work in partnership with others to achieve solutions valued by and beneficial to all.

Delimitations

In preparing this chapter, I bounded the topic in four ways:

I discuss dietetic practice in clinical settings. Readers may consider how or whether the ideas in this chapter have relevance for practice in other settings including community, public health, food service, private practice, academic, government, and others. While a reader may make connections to the concepts covered, it was not my intent to generalize the topic to make it widely applicable.

While there are many aspects one could explore about clinical nutrition practice using a critical social theory lens, I have examined forms of power including those that clinical dietitians have and may (perhaps unknowingly) have over others and those to which these workers are subject.

I have taken a post-oppositional view, that is, resisting challenges to power, not attempting to "one up" others. This relates to how clinical dietitians can recognize forms of power in their work settings and engage collaboratively toward optimizing relationships and environments to benefit those who work there and those who are residents, clients, or visitors.

Further to # 3, my interest is in identifying and enacting "the kind of help that helps" (Wilber 1993, p. 255) that is attainable and sustainable and produces optimal outcomes for all.

Ontology

The chapter is based on the values of client-centeredness and co-creation of the goals of nutritional care among clients, families, and health services personnel during times of illness, disability, and injury or at the end of life. The principle underpinning these values is the essentiality of the lived experiences of people who seek consultation with a dietitian or who find themselves in a dietitian's care (i.e., where nutritional care is a standard or requirement of care for a person with the client's diagnosis). To be relevant and appropriate, nutrition care planning and implementation, and nutrition education and counselling involve blending the experiences, preferences, and declared needs of clients and families with nutritional/medical standards of care. Lived experiences of patients, clients, and communities mingled with the learned experiences of practitioners and clinicians are integral to the co-production of knowledge that informs clinical nutrition practice.

Clinical Dietitians Having Power Over

Historical

In Canada and elsewhere in the developed world, dietitians have been recognized as healthcare service providers for about a century (Lang and Upton 1973). As such, they have status as regulated health professionals with "registered" status in the province in which the individual practices. While this is not consistent around the world, where there are such Acts in place, dietitians historically hold power conferred by government legislation. This means ready recognition of the registered dietitian (RD) or professional dietitian (PDt) credentials along with their obligations to protect the public from harm (e.g., Professional Dietitians Act, NS House of Assembly 2009).

Authority and Expertise

Registered dietitians working in clinical settings are recognized as members of a group with the power of expertise and positions as members of the healthcare team, and as those who hold university degrees and who have completed advanced practicum preparatory training in healthcare settings (a location that holds status in North America). In keeping with the biomedical model that forms the foundation for care provided in most clinical settings (i.e., the person is identified largely by the medical diagnosis and condition that he/she/they is/are living with), registered dietitians have professional knowledge of medical nutrition therapy and possess the legislated authority (NSDA 2018) to consult with other health professions about the care of another and to provide advice to others about the management of their bodies. Dietitians' socialization to have expert knowledge (MacLellan et al. 2011) is reinforced in many clinical settings. Diet prescriptions are routinely implemented, and clients are advised on what they *should* eat (e.g., in Snetselaar 2008), even when a diet prescription may not be entirely appropriate for the person's dietary needs, personal situation, or nutrition education needs and preferences (Morley et al. 2016).

Socioeconomic Status

The majority of dietitians are middle-income earners and, as such, have access to food and housing that includes kitchen facilities. Clients may have different income status and living conditions. Having access to kitchen facilities and food, having food storage and preparation knowledge and skills, and being able to read documents shared by a dietitian or from other sources (e.g., the Internet) are important considerations when planning nutritional care and offering advice and guidance. Where personal resources are limited, clients may not be in positions to implement nutritionc are recommendations (Morley et al. 2016).

Physical Arrangements

People receiving or seeking care in clinical settings are vulnerable compared to those providing care (Wartenberg 1991). The following is a partial description of the many ways one's sense of power and personal autonomy can be minimized in clinical settings.

People are often frightened or anxious being in unfamiliar surroundings where there is a lot of activity owing to the multiple and varied responsibilities of healthcare team members. One may be confused about what is happening related to their care in the moment and about what will happen. In clinical settings people (patrons/clients) are expected to have implicit trust in the health professionals who work there, and that these strangers possess specialized knowledge and will use it to aid the person seeking care.

People receiving care in institutions often feel unwell and may not be able to think clearly or to vocalize ideas, worries, and concerns. When they can do so, they may not feel heard. For some, owing to neurologic conditions, pain, or physical barriers, they may not be able to speak or to write out their thoughts. There are many interruptions and visits by physicians and staff members such that one's time is not one's own. Care provider visits may seem too short or infrequent for a person to feel assured they are getting the best or suitable care.

A person may be physically lower than care providers, for example, lying in a bed or on a stretcher or sitting in wheelchair so that care providers who are standing must literally be looked up to. Positionally, those who are higher vertically are considered to have more power such that these situations can be uncomfortable for people unable to stand (Wartenberg 1991). People receiving care may be in hospital gowns and robes or in their own pajamas, while health professionals are dressed in professional attire and uniforms or are wearing lab coats (a symbol of power). Sometimes healthcare workers wear masks, gloves, and gowns or use equipment that disguises their features. These are depersonalizing and can be unnerving when the appearance of those providing treatment and care is hidden or distorted. Being in these situations can reduce a person's sense of comfort and minimizes their sense of autonomy and power.

Dietitians are able to move throughout the facilities where they work, go "behind the scenes," confer with other members of the healthcare team, and access clients' personal files and institutional policy documents. They are also able to add to clients' medical files their nutrition assessment and care plan documents whereas, people seeking care do not have this privilege. What a dietitian records can influence future care provided by other dietitians and other health professionals.

Interpersonal Power

Drawing from my own experiences consulting health professionals, some dietitians may remain anonymous and not disclose their names or their purpose for the conversation. I have had to ask care providers for their names and the findings from their examinations, beyond passively accepting a prescription with the expectation that I would have it filled and would take it as prescribed. Partly, I wonder how health professionals can have such poor interpersonal skills. Further, I recognize the unwillingness to disclose as an action that places the power with those who do the withholding.

Decision-Making Power

Dietitians have power to participate in, advocate for, contribute to, and influence policy-related discussions pertaining to medical nutrition therapy. This can contribute to or hinder relationships between dietitians and clients and all care that a client receives from any care provider in the healthcare sector.

Dietitians working in clinical settings have authority to make decisions that affect the food and eating experiences of people who are receiving care. On one hand, dietitians are in positions to make diet prescriptions and to order what clients will receive for meals, tubefeedings, and, in some locations, parenteral nutrition. Depending on the culture of the facility in which a dietitian works, dietitians can exercise the power to restrict foods a client has requested or to add items to meal trays or snacks that the person did not request. Because tubefeedings and parenteral nutrition orders are outside of the knowledge of most people (whereas food is not), when a person is in a position to need this type of feeding, dietitians have complete power over what to order; clients are expected to have complete trust in the dietitian.

Organizational Structures

Organizational structures, an organization's mission statement and objectives, and the policies and procedures of the organization or department influence what a dietitian can do and what services they can offer in a given clinical setting. Sometimes these are inconsistent with clients' needs and preferences. For example, a client may wish to consult with a dietitian about ongoing difficulties eating as a result of medical treatments that happened years before. If an organizational policy states that only patients on active treatment or within 5 years of treatment can access dietitian services, people who have long-term challenges eating because of their treatments are not likely to be seen. A dietitian may decide to overlook the policy and provide care resulting in additional problems. In fee-for-service organizations, this can result in billing problems or (surprise) expenses for the client and may prevent others (for whom the policy was written) from accessing nutrition care. Ideally, such policies are evidence-based; however, some may be based on organizational history or values of efficiency and inputs/outputs, and not on care that reflects clients' real needs. Policies and guidelines require ongoing review and revision to incorporate new information about the long-term effects of medical treatments that affect eating. Clinical dietitians are important in creating or contributing to such policies to ensure they meet clients' ongoing needs and preferences.

Whose Voice Matters? Who Considers What as Important in Nutrition Care Management?

Consideration of the myriad factors that influence a person's life and well-being is foundational to providing client-centered nutritional care. Healthcare professionals, sometimes without being aware of it, can exercise power over clients by not paying attention to or not considering social, economic, and other factors that will affect how people will manage to feed themselves when they return home. It may happen that nutrition care in clinical settings is so focused on maintaining physical health or physiologic balance that other aspects of nutrition assessment are overlooked, minimized, or ignored. Obvious considerations when planning for long-term personal nutrition care are whether a person can afford to obtain food (Green et al. 2008; Williams et al. 2012), and, if so, are they safe to do so, and can they safely store, prepare, and eat food and maintain food preparation area cleanliness to prevent foodborne illness (Elaun 2018)?

Emotional connections with and through food are fundamental to eating and may not always relate to health condition management (Morley et al. 2016). For example, endeavouring to maintain *normal* family meals or food preparation roles may be more important to a person than to attend to their prescribed diet or nutrition recommendations. For people in these situations, family harmony and pleasure are more important than any potential negative consequences of not eating as advised. For some, care of animals and pets, their business, being able to pay bills, or other daily activities take precedence over self-care. Ideally, health professionals create conditions to witness clients' concerns about eating when outside of the clinical setting so that any possible barriers to eating to manage health conditions can be discussed and solutions thought through.

Some people are afraid to eat when responsible for managing their own food intake; this may be to avoid pain that follows eating or fear of making a mistake and "not eating right." It is important to witness and respect these concerns and to continue to offer support or to find valid, acceptable, and reliable referral sources. One of the problems in many parts of Canada, and perhaps elsewhere, is that there are few to no community-based nutrition services (such as visiting dietitians or home care dietitians). Therefore, when dietitians in clinical settings make referrals to community nutrition services, they must ensure that such services exist in their area and that there is continuity of care between the clinical and home settings (Dietitians of Canada 2016).

All of the examples highlight the integral nature of the client's voice in planning for and implementing nutrition care. This calls for an examination of whether or how one exercises one's power over clients and their family care partners.

Clinical Dietitians and Being Powered Over

As with considering the forms of power that dietitians may hold, reflecting on the ways that dietitians may be powered over cannot be viewed as universal and experienced by all clinical dietitians in exactly the same way. In preparing this section of the chapter, I reflected on Wartenberg's *Forms of Power* (1991) and considered how some of these may be enacted in the workplaces of clinical dietitians.

I was privileged in the years I worked as a clinical dietitian and clinical nutrition manager to have physician, nursing, and other coworkers who not only valued nutrition care in the overall medical management of the people for whom we provided care; these colleagues valued us as individuals whom they trusted unreservedly. Not all dietitians are so fortunate.

Historical

The roles of clinical dietitians have changed immensely since the dietetics profession came into being. In the early years of dietitians working in hospitals (Brady 2017), dietitians unquestioningly followed physicians' diet orders. In some cases, dietitians prepared foods for 'special diets' (foods modified in some way that the cooks were not able to prepare when focusing on large-scale food production). More often today, dietitians respond to 'Dietitian To See' orders or screen or assess every person admitted to hospital with particular diagnoses (per Standards of Care or Standards of Practice for the facility). In many facilities, clinical dietitians have control over medical nutrition therapy planning and administration. Clinical dietitians work collaboratively with all other team members (physicians, nurses, rehabilitation therapists, social workers, pharmacists, etc.) to ensure that nutritional care aligns with the overall goals of care for the person's hospitalization or treatment.

This is the ideal; not all dietitians will find that they work in this situation. Where team members did not have any nutrition teaching in their own training or were educated by instructors who were not up to date on evidence about the value of nutritional support, dietitians may encounter antiquated views of their roles. They may find that nutrition is not considered relevant in plans for overall care (as short-cited and unbelievable as this is since no one can regain health or physiologic stability without sustenance) (Allard et al. 2015).

Sex Demographics

Between 95% and 100% of dietitians in Canada (depending on the province or territory) identify as female (Dietitians of Canada 2011). The predominance of women as dietitians has been consistent since the profession shifted in the early twentieth century from a medical specialty[1] to that requiring preparatory education in home economics and registration with a provincial dietetics association or college (Lang and Upton 1973). As of 2016, up to 5% of Canadian dietitians identify as male, a change from the early twentieth century (Gheller and Lordly 2015). In contrast, the sex demographics of physicians in Canada have changed dramatically in this same time period. "Women have gone from accounting for just seven per cent of physicians in 1970 to more than 40 per cent today" (Ciolfe 2017). In 2017, 60% of physicians under the age of 35 are identified as female (compared to 52% of those in the 35–44-year group, 43% in the 45–54-year age group, 35.5% in the 55–64-year group, and 20% in the 65+ group) (Canadian Medical Association 2017). This indicates that more women are entering into medical practice. It is interesting to consider what difference, if any, these differences in sex demographics among dietitians

---

[1] Until about 1900, *dieticians* (with a "c") were gentlemen physicians who prescribed diet therapy before effective surgical and infection control therapies were developed (Morley 2018).

and physicians have on practice settings. Are they more egalitarian, the same, or something else? No extant literature on this topic was located. What has been studied are physicians' perceptions of power, with encounters with patients, not with healthcare team members.

Nimmon and Stenfors-Hayes (2017) found three types of responses when physicians were asked about their power in patient-physician encounters. One group reported that their superiority in patient-physician encounters was appropriate because patients had to trust the physicians' knowledge and skills. Another group reported that their power was waning (patients questioned their decisions), and a third group felt that power was not relevant to how they practiced owing largely to their personalities and interests in shared decision-making. How these findings might be relevant to power relationships among healthcare team members has not been studied.

The sex demographics question remains: How, if at all, does having more women as physicians affected power relationships in healthcare teams, including those between physicians and dietitians? The relevance of these findings for clinical dietitians is that long-standing patriarchal power dynamics in healthcare settings may benefit from having more women as physicians. This assumes however, that these newer-to-practice physicians bring a gender-neutral perspective to their work and do not replicate hierarchies (of position and sex) of the past.

Hierarchical

In any clinical setting, organizational charts outline who reports to whom. Clinical dietitians may report to a senior dietitian or a manager, director, or program lead who may be a dietitian, registered nurse, physician, or some other health and human services professional. This person, in turn, reports to an administrator responsible for clinical services who reports to the senior administrator, who reports to a board. Clinical dietitians become adept at knowing to what level they have decision-making authority and when they need approval from those in positions higher up in the organizational structure. In addition, clinical dietitians are learning of the importance of sharing successes, achievements, and external recognitions (e.g., awards, prizes, grants, fellowship, working group invitations) with senior personnel so that these accomplishments and milestones do not go unnoticed in the organization. Further, these milestones can serve as evidence to support future requests to senior administration for resources or approvals to proceed with a program, service, or research idea.

Meanwhile, other health professionals have their own reporting hierarchies. Physicians may have admitting privileges yet are not employees of the healthcare facility, whereas hospitalist physicians would be employees. As such, they would also have a reporting hierarchy to which they are responsible. These various reporting routes can be, and often are, in competition with each other for resources. Dietitians, because their departments or services are smaller than those of nursing, pharmacy, or rehabilitation services, tend to have less influence than the larger (more highly funded) services.

Advocates

While clinical dietitians determine the nutrition care to be provided to a person receiving treatment at clinical facilities, systems factors influence whether and what amount of nutritional care can be offered. In Canada, senior administrators determine the budgets for dietitians' positions and advocate with provincial or territorial governments for any additional funding when there is interest in expanding clinical nutritional services. The role of senior administrators in advocacy on behalf of clinical dietitians' services builds on the previous suggestion to make administrators aware of the activities, successes, and needs of clinical nutrition services to encourage and prepare them to pitch proposals for funding. Consequently, the systematic gathering of formative and summative evaluations of clinical nutrition services will yield the information to report to senior administrators. This includes numeric information (e.g., number of participants/consultations) as well as client perspectives on what the service did for or meant to them and their families. An example of how this might be accomplished is to use the Clients' Perceptions about Nutrition Counseling (CPNC) instrument (Morley-Hauchecorne et al. 1994). The CPNC was developed to be used to generate quantitative results on what counselling was provided and client perceptions of how well the information/support they received addressed their needs, as well as client insights about and comments on the services. Results from the administration of the instrument have been used by clinical dietitians and managers for quality improvement of services and by senior dietitians to advocate for maintaining or expanding clinical nutrition services (e.g., Cook et al. 2006; Cai 2017; Noddin 2017).

Recognizing and Working with Forms of Power

When working as a clinical dietitian, either having power over or being powered over, recognizing and naming the forms of power operating within one's workplace can serve as a starting place for discussions with students, dietitians, and coworkers about issues of power and privilege that is conferred when one holds professional status. In terms of having power, sorting through these forms of power can aid clinical dietitians' understandings of how they might embrace client-centeredness in their practice to work in partnership with others. A simple example is considering the terms used in referring to the people for whom dietitians offer nutrition care. The word *patient* is inherently passive, meaning "receiving or registered to receive medical treatment" (Oxford Dictionary Online, 2018). Further, language can depersonalize as when referring to a person in terms of their condition, e.g., *celiac* or *diabetic*. Clinical dietitians can consider the terms they can use that reflect how they want to work in collaboration to balance power.

For clinical dietitians, conversations about having power and being powered over can illuminate the ways that both forms of power affect the work they do and the work they might wish to be doing. From a post-oppositional view, appreciating forms of power is not about endeavouring to 'take' or 'have' more of it. Instead, one can recognize how power supports what they are doing and how they can create conditions to continue that support. This may include sharing insights with those who are or who could be advocates.

Importantly, recognizing forms of power invites consideration of how one might benefit others by leveraging one's own power to support another's position or concerns while not 'taking over'.

Closing

As I wrote this chapter, detailing forms of power I have experienced when I worked as a clinical dietitian and from talking to colleagues about their work in this area, I observed that the forms of power I could identify that dietitians held outnumbered those where dietitians were powered over. I wondered if this was because of the types of positions I have held, the workplace cultures where I worked, the people who worked there, or something else? Was it because I worked in places where the Food and Nutrition Services directors had advocated for clinical nutrition with senior administration? Was it our (my fellow dietitians and my) commitment to the essentiality of nutrition care and nutritional support even though some healthcare colleagues might not have agreed or were not interested? In Canada, Schools or Departments of nutrition and dietetics in universities are not always associated with health sciences thereby, Nutrition students are not always invited to participate in on-campus interprofessional training. As a result, graduates of other health professions (non-dietitians) may not be familiar with the roles, responsibilities, and qualities of dietitians and may carry this lack of awareness into their practice. This calls upon dietitians to advocate for their inclusion and participation in the health care team.

Exploration of the forms of power that influence clinical nutrition practice revealed the following commonalities. First, both having power as a clinical dietitian and being powered over have their roots in history. Power dynamics in workplaces are not new, and they often shift. Second, relationships with others are important to enhance the effectiveness of workplace activities and the results of offering care. Where there are power imbalances and where the ideal is to work in client-centered collaboration, workplace satisfaction and effectiveness are likely to suffer. Power is disrupted when the lived experiences of all people involved in caring relationships are valued and integral to how clinical dietitians approach their work.

Assignment

At ward rounds, a nurse asks you (the clinical dietitian) how compliant one of the patients is with their low-sodium diet prescription. Outline and describe the forms of power imbedded in this statement. Describe actions one might take in this situation.

A surgeon who is a member of a large multigenerational family of physicians who have worked for decades at the hospital (a wing is named after them) writes an order for a dietitian to see a patient before discharge for a weight-loss diet. The person for whom the consultation was ordered is surprised when they meet you, not knowing that the surgeon thought their weight was an issue. Outline and describe the forms of power imbedded in this statement. Describe actions one might take in this situation.

Your friend, a fellow intern/practicum student, came to you with concerns about an incident that deeply troubled her. She had been working that day with the outpatient dietitian. A trans woman, Susan, came in for information about transitioning and redistribution of body fat. The dietitian insisted on using the 'he' pronoun and using her legal name, David. The intern was seeking your help to deconstruct what happened as she could not figure out why she felt so upset. Outline and describe the forms of power imbedded in this statement. Describe actions one might take in this situation.

Definitions of Keywords and Terms

Forms of power	Forms of power refer to the many ways that power is a factor in social relationships. These include one's position within an organization; historical contribution(s) (of oneself or one's family members); expertise or authority; serving as a funding decision-maker (deciding who or what projects get funded and by how much); determining who has decision-making authority (including who has a voice, to what voices to attend, and how messages will be conveyed); one's personal or one's group's physical force or strength; gender; wealth; recognition and notoriety; and positional power (e.g., the teacher/student relationship) (Wartenberg 1991).
Post-oppositional perspective	Ways of working and engaging that move beyond being in opposition, that is, working collaboratively rather than counter to whomever or whatever one considers as the antagonist. Working from a post-oppositional perspective, one embraces

interconnectivity and creates conditions for fruitful dialogues toward transformational possibilities. One considers political, ethical, social, spiritual, intellectual, and pedagogical dimensions of issues. Keating (2013) declared that post-oppositionality "calls for and enacts innovative, radically inclusionary ways of reading, teaching, and communicating".

To be powered over	To be subject to the forms of power that another person or organization holds and wields.
To have power over	To exercise one's power over another or a group in a social relationship.

How This Chapter Addresses the Critical Dietetic Framework

The Critical Dietetics Framework is addressed in this chapter through the naming and discussion of forms of power that are inherent in all human communications and social situations including those occurring in clinical nutrition practice. Integrating the concepts of *power over* and b*eing powered over*, in addition to inviting consideration of a post-oppositional perspective, disrupts the view that clinical nutrition practice involved only a simple, clear-cut identification of a client's nutritional needs, the provision of meals and snacks consistent with these needs, and the making of nutrition information available so that people are able to feed themselves according to their diet prescriptions once in their own homes. Instead, the chapter was prepared to enhance awareness of the complex social environments and relationships extant in clinical practice settings, and that forms of power, a dietitian's own and those of others, influence all that happens in that work environment. Developing an understanding of what these relationships are and how they benefit some and not others may help clinical dietitians to recognize and explain the challenges they have encountered in learning how to contribute effectively to client care and the provision of clinical services.

The values grounding the chapter were client-centeredness, post-oppositionality, and the importance of relationship-building among clients, families, and health services personnel to recognize and address power differentials in the interest of client-identified optimal outcomes. To be relevant and appropriate, nutrition care planning is the coalescing of the experiences, preferences, and declared needs of clients and families with nutrition and medical standards of care. Socially just clinical nutrition practice is enhanced when the voices of all participants in clinical practice settings are heard, valued, and respected. The collective can collaborate to ensure that clinical nutrition services unquestionably benefit those for whom the services are intended. This requires some people to have a voice or a stronger voice and for others to recognize that for socially just needs to be met, the power they have held will redistribute.

References

Allard JP, Keller H, Jeejeebhoy K, Laporte M, Duerksen D, Gramlich L, Payette H, Bernier P, Vesnaver E, Davidson B, Teterina A, Lou W (2015) Malnutrition at hospital admission—contributors and effect on length of stay: a prospective cohort study from the Canadian malnutrition task force. J Parenter Enter Nutr. https://doi.org/10.1177/0148607114567902

Brady J (2017) Trading the apron for the white lab coat: A contemporary history of dietetics in Canada, 1954 to 2016. Doctoral thesis, Queen's University, Kingston

Cai C (2017). Development of an evaluation plan for nutrition counselling of orthopaedic prehabilitation programs in Nova Scotia Health Authority Western Zone. Acadia University Dietetic Practicum Research Project. Wolfville NS

Canadian Medical Association (2017) Physician Data Centre: Canadian physician statistics. Canadian Medical Association. Accessed 20 Apr 2018 at https://www.cma.ca/En/Pages/canadian-physician-statistics.aspx

Ciolfe T (2017, October 10) Female doctors are on the rise in Canada. Maclean's. Accessed 24 Apr 2018 at http://www.macleans.ca/news/canada/female-doctors-are-on-the-rise-in-canada/

Cook S, Nasser R, Comfort B, Larsen D (2006) Effect of nutrition counselling on client perceptions and eating behaviour. Can J Diet Pract Res 67(4):171–177. https://doi.org/10.3148/67.4.2006.171

Dietitians of Canada (2008) The need for a program of home-based nutrition services in British Columbia. Dietitians of Canada, Toronto

Dietitians of Canada (2011) The dietitian workforce in Canada meta-analysis report. Accessed 24 Apr 2018 at: http://www.dietitians.ca/Downloadable-Content/Public/Workforce-Meta-Analysis-Report-English-pdf.aspx

Dietitians of Canada (2016) Dietitians of Canada input to better Home Care in Canada consultation. Toronto: Dietitians of Canada. Accessed 21 Apr 2018 at: https://www.dietitians.ca/Dietitians-Views/Health-Care-System/Home-Care.aspx

Elaun S (2018) Field-testing the Nutrition Inventory for Community-Dwelling Elders (NICE) to determine consumer readability and comprehension. Honours thesis, School of Nutrition and Dietetics, Acadia University

Gheller B, Lordly D (2015) Males in dietetics, what can be learned from the nursing profession? A narrative review of the literature. Can J Diet Pract Res 76(4):166–171. https://doi.org/10.3148/cjdpr-2015-016

Green R, Williams PL, Blum I, Johnson CSJ (2008) Can Canadian seniors on public pensions afford a nutritious diet? Can J Aging 27(1):69–79

Keating A (2013) Transformation now! Toward a post-oppositional politics of change. University of Illinois Press, Champaign

Lang M, Upton E (1973) The dietetic profession in Canada. Canadian Dietetic Association, Toronto

MacLellan D, Lordly D, Gingras J (2011) Professional socialization in dietetics: a review of the literature. Can J Diet Pract Res 71:37–42

Morley C (2018) Dieticians and dietitians: exploring the evolution of practitioners and practices. Guest lecture, Mount St. Vincent University, March

Morley C, MacLellan D, Traviss K, Cividin T (2016) Developing an evidence-based framework and practice points for collaborative, client-centered nutrition education (3CNE). Can J Diet Pract Res 77:1–6

Morley-Hauchecorne C, Barr S, Sork T (1994) Evaluation of nutrition counselling in clinical settings: do we make a difference? J Am Diet Assoc 94(4):437–440

Nimmon L, Stenfors-Hayes T (2017) The "handling" of power in the physician-patient encounter: perceptions from experienced physicians. BMC Med Educ 16:114. https://doi.org/10.1186/s12909-016-0634-0

Noddin E (2017) Creation of an interview guide using the Value of Nutrition Education framework to assure the quality of the Diabetes Center 'Introduction to Diabetes' class. Acadia University Dietetic Practicum Research Project. Wolfville NS

Nova Scotia Dietetic Association (2018) About NSDA – Mission. At: https://nsdassoc.ca/public/about-nsda

Nova Scotia House of Assembly, Office of the Legislative Counsel (2009) Professional Dietitians Act. Government of Nova Scotia, Halifax

Snetselaar L (2008) Nutrition counseling skills for the nutrition care process. Jones and Bartlett Publishers, Sudbury

Wartenberg T (1991) Forms of power: from domination to transformation. Temple University Press, Philadelphia

Wilber K (1993) Grace and grit: spirituality and healing in the life and death of Treya Killam Wilber. Shambhala Press, Boston

Williams PL, MacAulay R, Anderson B, Barro K, Gillis DE, Johnson C et al (2012) "I would have never thought that I would be in such a predicament": voices from women experiencing food insecurity in Nova Scotia, Canada. J Hunger Environ Nutr (2–3):253–270

Chapter 6
Reshaping the Food System Using Food Democracy: Reorienting Consumer and Dietetic Practice

Sue Booth and John Coveney

Aims and Learning Outcomes

The aims of this chapter are twofold: firstly, to explore the practical roles and ways in which consumers may exert control over the current food system and foster alternative food systems and, secondly, to examine how dietetic practitioners may better support their clients and how as a profession they may operate as expert leaders to foster the development of healthier food systems and communities.

At the end of this chapter, readers (consumers and practitioners) will:

(i) Understand the nature and principles of democracy and how they may apply to food.
(ii) Understand what is wrong with the current industrial food system and how consumers may practice food democracy to exert control over the food system.
(iii) Gain knowledge about the shortcomings of traditional dietetic advice and strategies to empower and better equip consumers.
(iv) Understand and be able to apply new practice frameworks, which support civic dietetics and position dietetic practitioners as leaders in this space.

Summary

The industrial food system is broken, and this impacts on health, communities and local economies. Consumers can actively transform themselves into food citizens and exert control over 'Big Food'. Like citizens practising food democracy, dietetic

S. Booth (✉) · J. Coveney
Flinders University, Adelaide, SA, Australia
e-mail: sue.booth@flinders.edu.au; john.coveney@flinders.edu.au

© Springer Nature Switzerland AG 2019
J. Coveney, S. Booth (eds.), *Critical Dietetics and Critical Nutrition Studies*,
Food Policy, https://doi.org/10.1007/978-3-030-03113-8_6

practitioners can also be active food democrats but in a different way, namely, with their clients and as expert leaders. This chapter makes the link between civic agriculture and civic dietetics and supports a case to abandon 'nutritionism'. Then, drawing on the work of Stevenson et al. (2007) and Enderton et al. (2017), we propose a new framework for practitioners for systems leadership in civic dietetics. The framework consists of navigators, whistle-blowers and advocates.

Introduction

Social movements often arise in response to injustices and offer practical mechanisms for dialogue, new ways of thinking and galvanising people towards action that result in system change. Seminal movements such as the civil rights movement in America and the women's liberation movement have irrevocably changed the course of history, while newer movements such as Mothers Against Drunk Driving (MADD) and People for the Ethical Treatment of Animals (PETA) are incrementally exerting change and building community awareness. Food democracy and critical dietetics are both examples of movements that play an important role in fostering change. Importantly the need for these changes is coming from a belief that many of the current structures and processes are simply not working for the majority. For example, rise of alternative food movements such as 'slow', 'local', 'clean' or 'organic' all speak to people being dissatisfied with factory-farmed, ultra-processed industrial food and seeking alternatives.

Fundamentally, food democracy is a citizen protest, a social uprising in response to the globalisation and commodification of food. Using democratic processes, food democracy 'seeks to expose and challenge the anti-democratic forces of control and claim the rights and responsibilities of citizens to participate in decision making' (Hassanein 2003). Similarly, the critical dietetics movement was born out of practitioner discontent that many of the traditional approaches to nutrition were limited in their ability to reflect deeper meanings and the complexities of health and illness (Aphramor and Gingras 2009).

This chapter will introduce the food democracy and, by association, civic agriculture movements, which seek to empower consumers to reshape and influence the current food system for the better. Taking a critical dietetics perspective, we will argue that food democracy has practical application not only for consumers to exert more control on the food system but also for reorienting professional dietetic practice by incorporating a food system perspective where possible. Building on the work of Stevenson et al. (2007) and Enderton et al. (2017), we propose a new professional practice framework which includes three possible roles for dietetic practitioners to embrace: navigators, whistle-blowers and advocates.

What Is Food Democracy?

Food democracy can be considered a movement that seeks to create alternative food systems to improve health and transform passive consumers into active food citizens. Alternative food networks is a broad term which refers to new interconnections of food system actors that offer something different from the industrial food system or 'Big Food' as it is known.

Taking a system perspective, food democracy is a struggle between two opposing forces, namely, the industrial food system (representative of high levels of power and control) and food democracy/alternative food systems (representative of citizens trying to exert control to reshape the food system). In this 'David and Goliath' contest, food democracy provides a framework and tools for consumer efforts to loosen the industrial food system's vice-like grip on the food we eat and how the world is used.

Food democracy is a fledgling concept and the name is not always familiar. However everyday consumers are questioning the provenance and ethics of food in the current food system, particularly where new technologies such as nanotechnology are used. Questions often considered include: has this fresh produce been produced using chemical fertilisers and pesticides? Is this fish fillet from a sustainable fish species? Has this chicken been raised and slaughtered in accordance with animal welfare and ethical standards? Occasionally consumers are forced to ask questions about food safety when there have been food scares and scandals.

In a food democracy, everyday people use democratic processes such as openness and transparency, along with free and fair debate, to gather critical information about the food system and to ask probing questions of food corporations and others about production methods. In doing so, consumers start to gather and share information and empower themselves about where their food comes from and how they can respond meaningfully.

Driven by increasing environmental, social, ethical, health and food system concerns, some individuals and families are exerting their power and actively moving away from a reliance on industrially produced food. Food democracy can be practised at three different levels: individual/household, community and national.

(i) Food democracy at individual/household level

Essentially food democracy at the level of the home and the individual comprises making choices that allow the participants to be part of the actual process of producing food. At the level of the individual, this may be as specific as reskilling one's self for cooking and spending more time preparing food from 'scratch'. Or it could be using foods that are less likely to be using processes that will release large amounts of greenhouse gases and emphasising foods that are low on the food chain, with particular attention to fruits and vegetables. At the level of the household, it could mean growing food in a garden, a pot or a balcony. However small or insignificant this may appear to be, the important part is that it is a gesture towards taking back control.

(ii) Community-level food democracy

Community-level food democracy is essentially the joining together of efforts that help participants share the responsibility for growing and distributing food. This could mean farmers' markets, vegetable box schemes, food-sharing cooperatives and food swaps. In effect these activities constitute the building of alternative food systems and range in size and sophistication, e.g., farmers' market versus local food swap. The evidence for the increasing popularity of alternative systems, like farmers' markets, is compelling.

(iii) National-level food democracy

At the national level, food democracy can involve participants taking a more active role in the development of food policies and guidelines. The move from (a passive) consumer to (an active) citizen – or from consumer to prosumer – provides the opportunity to shape the food system, if even in a small way (Cruz. pers.comm. 17/4/18).

Consistent across these concepts of food democracy is the philosophy supported by Hassanein who suggests that food democracy 'is not only a goal or end point, additionally it's the *processes* used in achieving food democracy which are critical to our understanding of it' (Hassanein 2003). In other words, food democracy is not only about changing to an alternative food system but also being conscious of the processes by which the changes are being made. A good example here is the production of 'organic' foods that have been manufactured in large food processing plants. While the ingredients may themselves be 'organic', the overall philosophy is problematic because organic movements try to ensure that they have paid attention to the processes by which food is grown, not merely what is on the label.

The processes that Hassanein (2003) promotes are now captured in the idea of co-production of knowledge and action. Co-production challenges the ideas that there exists a body of expert knowledge that is passed down to non-experts who then put in place the advice they have been given. These models of the cascading effects of knowledge are now regarded to be limited in action and effects. Instead, the idea of shared expertise is cherished. This can be summarised by the idea that experts have 'learned experience' by virtue of them having to learn about and reproduce ideas as part of their expert practices. But this can only go so far; 'learned experience' needs to be accompanied by 'lived experience' which comes from the everyday quotidian knowledge that resides in the individuals and communities with whom experts work. Thus the combination of 'learned experience' and 'lived experience' is a potent basis for working together respectfully and with the possibilities that the basis of knowledge of each is valued. Co-production is now part of some clinical practices and community participation in public service decision-making.

Civic Agriculture

It has been suggested that civic agriculture brings together production and consumption activities with communities and offers consumers alternatives to the commodities produced, by large food manufacturers (Lyson 2004). Sociologist Thomas

Lyson conceived the term civic agriculture to describe 'the emergence and growth of community-based agriculture and food production activities that not only meet consumer demands for fresh, safe, and locally produced foods but create jobs, encourage entrepreneurship, and strengthen community identity' (Lyson 1999, p. 2).

In practice, civic agriculture can take the form of consumers having a more active role in the food supply chain, which they use. For example, community-supported agriculture (CSA) projects often take the form of cooperatives where food producers and community members work together to understand and appreciate each other's needs. Moreover, it is common in these arrangements for community members to become share- or stakeholders in the farms and thus actively involved in the 'on-farm' production of the food which they will eventually consume.

Why Do We Need Food Democracy, and What's Wrong with the Current Food System?

Remaking the food system suggests neither revolution nor a radical transformation but rather deliberate, sometimes unsophisticated multipronged opportunistic, consistent effort. Hamilton (2005) argues that there is no revolution in seeking better food or wanting more information, rather food democracy is about restoring something which we should have today (Hamilton 2005).

Eating is a highly political act, and the realms of food democracy and alternative agri-food networks are highly politicised spaces. An examination of democratic theory by Barber (2004) suggests some types of democracy may be more effective than others. 'Thin democracy' is rooted in an individualistic 'rights' frame that diminishes the role of citizens in democratic governance. Democratic values are provisional, optional and conditional resulting in limited citizen participation, public good or civic virtue outcomes (Barber 2004). The more favourable alternative is 'strong democracy' (Barber 2004) which embraces a vision of politics that can respond to and adapt to the changing world. Strong democracy is characterised by people self-governing as much as possible rather than delegating their power and responsibilities. Applying this concept to food democracy, practising 'strong democracy' is a way of living that supports engagement, active participation and empowerment of the community in [food] decisions that affect them.

Alternative food movements encompass two forms of political activity (Scrinis 2007). Firstly, oppositional politics encompasses activities directly opposing or challenging existing institutions, structures and practices as a way of stimulating new developments within the existing food system. Oppositional politics often centres on a single issue, but encompassing a broader food system critique, with the goal of reforming government policies, corporate power and practices or safety regulations. An example is consumer protests by members of the Australian Food Sovereignty Alliance against a 2018 decision by the Food Standards Australia New Zealand (FSANZ) to approve the sale of genetically modified Golden Rice.

Secondly, constructivist politics and activities seek to create new food systems despite the 'Big Food' behemoth. They foster 'hotbeds' of innovation underpinned by democratic processes, for example, the inner city Perth farm that grows leafy greens for restaurants and gives work to the unemployed. In building a new food model, the Green World Revolution addresses both social and environmental issues, namely, underutilised urban spaces and youth unemployment.

Warriors, Builders and Weavers

Local food system experts claim that citizen involvement in food systems supports local economies, improves human health and leads to healthier communities and environments. Food system actors are an increasing group of citizens concerned with developments in the agri-food system. Other frameworks conceptualise more clearly change activities in the food system and the role that individual actors may play (Stevenson et al. 2007). Stevenson et al. (2007) suggest three main goals of change activities: (i) *inclusion* which is about increasing citizen participation, (ii) *reformation* which aims to alter food system operating guidelines for the better and (iii) *transformation* where food systems undergo transformation into new models of operation. Key citizen actors within the food system space may adopt three possible strategic orientations or roles to stimulate possible change activities. These roles are 'warrior', 'builder' and 'weaver'. However, it should be noted that these roles are not mutually exclusive. 'Warrior' work is about resistance, seeking to create political pressure and recruit and mobilise others for action. The goal of 'warrior' work is to stimulate change and to highlight concerns to others. In many ways, 'warrior' work is similar to Scrinis's (2007) 'oppositional' politics; it is adversarial, public and political. A good example of 'warrior' work is that undertaken by *MAdGE* (Mothers Against Genetic Engineering in Food and the Environment). *MAdGE*, along with other pockets of resistance from scientific and community groups, emerged in response. *MAdGE* has been most active in Australia where it has harassed the Victorian state government, especially when a moratorium on banning the growing GM canola for commercial purposes was lifted. *MAdGE* has also engaged in acts of civil disobedience in supermarkets where members have targeted and relabeled food products suspected of harbouring GM ingredients with stickers proclaiming 'contaminated – genetically modified'. The ensuing publicity has given greater voice to *MAdGE* which now sees itself as a campaign where 'Mothers are Demystifying Genetic Engineering' (Booth et al. 2018).

'Builder' work focuses on creating new or alternative food systems; it is highly entrepreneurial and risky, rather than political and adversarial. The main focus of builders is on starting and sustaining new agri-food businesses (Stevenson et al. 2007). For example, community-supported agriculture (CSA) is a sustainable food production system where small farmers on the urban fringes sell direct to consumers. Sometimes referred to as 'CSA box schemes', they offer a direct relationship model with efficient and transparent supply chains for fresh produce. Consumers subscribe for 6–12 months of the farm's growing season and receive a weekly box of fresh produce delivered. In the CSA business model, there is no retailer involved, and producers are better able to respond to consumer feedback. 'Builders' in CSAs may include small local farmers, volunteers, subscribers, neighbours and all those involved in the supporting model.

'Weaver' work involves connection, both inter- and intra-sectoral linkages between people and food system actors (Stevenson et al. 2007). For example, in a farmer's market, 'weaver' work may be performed by the market manager, public relations staff and the communications manager. These actors build sophisticated linkages both internally and externally. Within a farmer's market, they foster communication between stallholders, members, customers and the management committee. Externally activities undertaken by 'weavers' include liaison with local councils, seeking media coverage and publicity, updating websites and social media profiles and meeting with sponsors, tourism and cultural representatives, festival organisers and local businesses. All of these 'weaver' functions serve to enhance the farmer's market profile and to ensure the successful operation of the weekly market.

'Shepherding' Community Engagement

'Shepherding' is a type of systems leadership; it is 'an intentional process of fostering trust, connecting food system actors, tracking readiness and making strategic requests to help interested community members define food system roles for themselves' (Enderton et al. 2017). In the context of a multicomponent, multi-stakeholder local food system collaboration in Northeast Iowa, 'shepherds' are paid staff. Paid professionals acting as 'shepherds' are important because they bring expertise, formal legitimacy and organisational support (Enderton et al. 2017).

Although 'shepherding' may infer guiding or directing people in a particular direction, this is not the case in this example. 'Shepherds' help others in the community to choose what is important and determine which direction to go (Enderton et al. 2017). 'Shepherding' encompasses listening, building networks and relationships, strategic guiding and nudging to help key stakeholders or community members to commence activities or expand their roles (Enderton et al. 2017). Efforts to rebuild food systems encompass co-leadership between both community/citizen involvement and leadership ('grass roots') and professional experts ('grass tops').

Reorienting Dietetic Practice

It has been argued that critical dietetics "...proposes broadening our lens beyond traditional/dominant paradigms and embracing new ways of framing how we research, educate and practice in dietetics..." (Aphramor and Gingras 2009). This section will examine the intersection of critical dietetics and food democracy in strengthening dietetic practice and empowering clients.

A fundamental premise underpinning dietetic practice and the promulgation of dietary advice is what is termed 'nutritionism', that is, 'a view of nutrients as biochemical entities that are independent of cultural, environmental and bodily processes' (Scrinis 2008). Implicit in this biomedical approach is a reductionist view of nutrients and the role they play in physical health on influencing individual behaviour change and modifying health. 'Nutritionism' limits professional scope resulting in consumers trying to implement practical dietary advice within the context of an overwhelmingly complex food system, also known as 'Big Food' (Hamilton 2004).

Since the 1980s calls have been made for the profession to move beyond 'nutritionism' and embrace food system and sustainability issues. Combining the power of critical dietetics and food democracy offers ways to re-examine 'nutritionism' with the view to honing dietetic practice to be more relevant to contemporary food systems and consumers.

Practising Civic Dietetics

Civic agriculture is an important facet of food democracy. Practitioners who understand civic agriculture and integrate local food system knowledge into dietary advice extend the boundaries of practice beyond 'nutritionism'. Complex food systems have a considerable impact on communities, health and the environment and warrant a more sophisticated level of dietary advice about food choices that dietitians will be expected to provide (Wilkins et al. 2010). This reorientation of the dietetic practice and alignment with the values of civic agriculture is known as 'civic dietetics'. In practice, civic dietetics is the application of dietetics to enhance public health by addressing food system structures, impacts and policies and their relationship to food choices (Wilkins et al. 2010).

In the United States, integration of civic dietetics and sustainable food system approaches has included the integration of food system and sustainability concepts into some dietetics intern training programs and the establishment of the *Journal of Hunger and Environmental Nutrition* and its associated practice group. The latter has been described as leaders in promoting and integrating food system sustainability into the dietetic profession. However, critics have argued a reason for the slow uptake of civic dietetics may be indicative of the strength of their alliances with the food industry.

In Australia, the practice of civic dietetics is a relatively unknown concept. With the growth of food and critical dietetics movements, and consumer interest in food provenance, it is timely for civic dietetics to emerge. It is timely too for dietetic practice settings to embrace the idea of co-production, mentioned earlier in the chapter. The attention to 'learned experience' of experts in the technical aspect of an issue or problem and the 'lived experience' patients and the communities who are expected to benefit from the systems in which we work provides a strong foundation for collaborative partnerships.

A New Framework: Navigators, Whistle-Blowers and Advocates

Having considered both Stevenson et al. (2007) and Enderton et al.'s (2017) frameworks and roles of food system actors (both citizens and paid professionals) to foster food system change, we propose a new systems leadership framework for the dietetic profession. Implicit in this framework is Enderton's concept of dietitians operating as paid professionals, namely, 'grass tops', working with consumers interested in 'grass-roots' activism and leadership. This framework is cognisant of civic dietetics and the roles of practitioners in aligning their practice with a leadership role in food system change. The three main roles are:

(i) Navigators

Like Enderton et al.'s 'shepherds', civic dietitians are well positioned to help consumers navigate the food system. In practice this may include providing information, critical skills and tools to eaters about the industrial and alternative food systems and the public health impacts. Digital platforms including online courses, mobile phone apps and e-learning opportunities provide increased information access for geographically isolated or busy consumers.

(ii) Whistle-Blowers

A whistle-blower is a person who exposes any kind of information or activity that is deemed illegal, unethical or not correct within an organisation that is either private or public. As experts in food and food systems, dietitians have the legitimacy to publically comment on instances of food crime that is immoral or illegal practices in the food industry. Food crimes may include adulteration of foods, substitution or contamination which may impact on human health as well as fraudulent or illegal practices. Food crimes such as the 2008 Chinese powdered milk scandal involving the substitution of melamine and the subsequent worldwide implications would be situations worthy of commentary.

(iii) Advocates

Dietitians are the peak profession dealing with food and diet-related disease. The national peak body, Dietitians Association of Australia, already advocates for a better health system, improvements in public health and reducing the consumption of diets high in fat, salt and sugar. However consideration should be given to further embrace their collective power as a profession and form a *global* alliance advocating for a better food system. Globally professionals such as doctors, nurses and lawyers are involved in groups calling for an end to gun control, nuclear weapons, conflict and civil war and gender-based violence. These advocacy groups demand considerable global attention to issues of injustice and place political pressure on governments to enact policy change.

The role of a global professional nutrition alliance may include advocating for healthier alternative food systems, calling for an end to food crimes, improved regulations and public health.

Conclusion

The aims of this chapter were to examine ways in which ordinary people may exert control over the current food system and foster alternative food systems. It also sought to explore how dietitians can advise and equip their clients and communities to be genuine collaborators. These aspects of dietetic practice will not always sit comfortably for those who have been trained to believe they have special wisdom that is theirs and only they can pass on to others, nor will it be easy for associations who are often riding professional boundaries to bolster the credibility of members. However, dietitians have much to gain, and little to lose, by considering their role as more participative partners with individuals and communities with which they work.

Assignment/Discussion Questions

1. 'Big Food' behaving badly.
   Our industrial food system is broken. Research and select a recent news item exposing an example of an industrial 'food crime'.

   - How has this incident come about and what factors may have contributed?
   - What might be the motivation for industrial 'food crimes'?
   - What might be some public health ramification of 'food crimes'?

2. A Tale of Two Food Systems.
   Compare and contrast an example of the industrial food system (such as a large national supermarket chain or global food company) with an example of food democracy in practice (such as a local farmer's market).

   - What do you notice about the types of food sold in each example?
   - What are the elements of 'democracy' in each system such as transparency of information and free and open discussion?
   - Consider how easy it is to navigate each of these systems to purchase food if you had a chronic condition such as diabetes.

Definition of Keywords and Terms

Big food	Refers to the transnational food and beverage industry that is powerful, profit driven and focussed on the manufacture of ultra-processed foods with serious consequences for public health and the environment.
Civic agriculture	"The emergence and growth of community-based agriculture and food production activities that not only meet consumer demands for fresh, safe, and locally produced foods but create jobs, encourage entrepreneurship, and strengthen community identity" (Lyson 1999, p. 2).
Civic dietetics	Civic Dietetics is the application of dietetics to enhance public health by addressing food system structures, impacts and policies and their relationship to food choices (Wilkins et al. 2010).
Food crime	Activities encompassing economic deception and physical harms, issues of personal health and fraudulent activities such as food substitution, adulteration, and mis-representation (Croall 2007).
Food democracy	Food democracy is the counterweight to the industrial food system. It can be considered a movement that seeks to create alternative food systems to improve health and transform passive consumers into active food citizens.
Nutritionism	A view of "nutrients as biochemical entities that are independent of cultural, environmental and bodily processes" (Scrinis 2008).

How the Chapter Addresses the Critical Dietetics Framework

This chapter aligns with the proposed critical dietetics framework in two main ways. Firstly, an appreciation of multidisciplinary and trans-theoretical approaches to understanding food, health and people. Implicit in the very title of this chapter is a scene of interdisciplinary scholarship and a cross-section of theoretical approaches, which add to the richness of the examination. Starting with the term "food democracy", we have the intersection of the world of food with that of political science. At first glance, these might at first seem unlikely companions, but as this chapter will explain, food democracy is quintessentially about consumers using democratic principles to regain some influence over the current industrial food system. In terms of broader food governance, food democracy is a way of decentralising control from "Big Food" and placing the locus of control back in the hands of the people. Here "Big Food" is taken to mean those large, often multinational, food companies which control the majority of food processes, food products and food choices in western jurisdictions but increasingly in other countries. The commodification of food and the resulting global food system is indeed a complex beast, with many players and actors. This chapter will delve into the realms of political science and explore the intersection of food with democratic principles, strong democracy and oppositional and constructivist politics.

Secondly, this chapter subscribes to the belief that policy and practice positions should be socially just. According to Lang, a core premise of food democracy is the public good, namely, that ecological and public health will be improved by democratic process (Lang 2007). This chapter will also explore the roles for dietetic and nutrition practitioners to move beyond nutrient-based advice and encompass a broader vision of the whole food system and the greater public or food system 'good' when working with clients. This reorientation of dietetic practice and alignment with the values of food democracy is known as civic dietetics.

References

Aphramor L, Gingras J (2009) That remains to be said: disappeared feminist discourses on fat in dietetic theory and practice. In: Rothblum ED, Solovay S (eds) Fat studies reader. New York Press, New York

Barber B (2004) Strong democracy: participatory politics for a new age. University of California Press, Berkeley

Booth S, Coveney J, Paturel D (2018) Countercrimes and food democracy: Suspects and citizens in remaking the food system. In: Gray A, Hinch R (eds) A handbook of food crime. Policy Press, Bristol

Croall H (2007) 'Food Crime', in P. Beirne and N. South (eds) Issues in green criminology: Confronting harms against environments, human and other animals, Portland, Oregon: Willan Publishing, pp 206–29

Enderton E, Bregendahl C, Topaloff A (2017) Shepherding community engagement to strengthen the local food system in Northeast Iowa. J Agric Food Syst Community Dev 7(2):85–100

Hamilton N (2004) Essay – food democracy and the future of American values. Drake J Agri 9:9–32

Hamilton N (2005) Food democracy II – revolution or restoration? J Food L Pol'y 1(1):13–42

Hassanein N (2003) Practicing food democracy: a pragmatic politics of transformation. J Rural Stud 19:77–86

Lang T (2007) Food security or food democracy? Pesticide News 78:12–16

Lyson TA (1999) Civic agriculture: reconnecting farm, food and community. University Press of New England, Hanover

Lyson TA (2004) Civic agriculture: reconnecting farm, food and community. Tufts University Press, Medord

Scrinis G (2007) From techno-corporate food to alternative agri-food movements. Local Global 4:112–140

Scrinis G (2008) On the idea of nutritionism. Gastronomica 8(1):39–48

Stevenson G, Ruhl K, Lezberg S, Clancy K (2007) Warrior, builder and weaver work. In: Hinrichs C, Lyson TA (eds) Remaking the North American Food System: strategies for sustainability. University of Nebraska, Lincoln

Wilkins J, Lapp J, Tagtow A, Roberts S (2010) Beyond eating right: the emergence of civic dietetics to foster health and sustainability through food system change. J Hunger Environ Nutr 5:2–12

Chapter 7
Critical Dietetics and Sustainable Food Systems

Liesel Carlsson, Kaye Mehta, and Clare Pettinger

Aims of Chapter and Learning Outcomes

In this chapter, we invite readers to consider a food system that is based on values where individual health, the health of the society (social system) and ecosystem health are of equal importance. With this as a lens, there is a clear need to move beyond the biosciences to consider transdisciplinary approaches as important for nutrition and dietetics in today and tomorrow's reality.

This chapter begins by briefly highlighting historical engagement of the nutrition and dietetics community with food system sustainability, before moving to define foundational concepts of sustainability in food systems and diets, from a systems perspective. It then provides some examples of how some of today's pressing nutritional challenges are sustainability challenges and examples of the interface between today's dietetics and food system sustainability. This chapter ends with a discussion on the role of nutrition and dietetic practitioners in food system sustainability and the needs and challenges for dietetic education to support that role.

At the end of this chapter, readers should be able to:

(i) Clearly understand the concept of sustainable food systems (SFS).
(ii) Describe some emerging roles for nutrition and dietetic professionals in contributing to food system sustainability.

L. Carlsson (✉)
Acadia University, Wolfville, NS, Canada
e-mail: liesel.carlsson@acadiau.ca

K. Mehta
Flinders University, Adelaide, SA, Australia

C. Pettinger
School of Health Professions (Faculty of Health and Human Sciences), University of Plymouth, Plymouth, UK

© Springer Nature Switzerland AG 2019
J. Coveney, S. Booth (eds.), *Critical Dietetics and Critical Nutrition Studies*,
Food Policy, https://doi.org/10.1007/978-3-030-03113-8_7

(iii) Consider engaging in deeper levels of inquiry about our responsibilities as a profession.

A Brief History of Sustainability in Dietetics

Issues of sustainability are not new to dietetics. One of the earliest (and best documented) "ecological nutritionists" was Ellen Swallow Richards. Richards was an early (human) ecologist, born in 1842. She worked as a chemist on issues such as water quality during an industrializing era and concerned herself with how that impacted public health. Richards was perhaps one of the first in North America to use the term "ecology", which "[she] saw as… neatly capturing her broad concerns for human-created environmental conditions and the health consequences for people living in those conditions" (Dyball and Carlsson 2017). As a woman in her day, despite a long career as a chemist, she was persuaded to throw passions for ecology into the domestic sciences, later called home economics, focusing more on managing the economy (a term with Greek roots meaning "household management") of the home. Subsequently, in many academic institutions, home economics evolved into the science of nutrition and dietetics, progressing from a practical focus on managing food as a family resource to an increasingly biomedical focus on the interrelationship between nutrients, health and disease.

Richards' ecological systems approach to home economics lays the groundwork for what Rebrovick would call "eco-dietetics" (Rebrovick 2015) or a dietetics that concerns itself with the interactions between eating and environmental, social, economic and political systems and celebrating food for the pleasure it provides. Here we briefly cover some central contributions to the emergence of an eco-dietetics discourse before unpacking some terms and key concepts.

In 1986, two American dietitians, Gussow and Clancy, proposed dietary guidelines for sustainability (Gussow and Clancy 1986). While this is often referred to as a pivotal publication proposing sustainability within the remit of dietetics, it reflected decades of civic activism on the responsibility of eaters to consider ecological sustainability. Though the ideas Gussow and Clancy put forth certainly did not lie dormant, biomedically driven dietetics dominated the focus of the profession for the following 20 years and, arguably, still does so today. In 2005, a framework referred to as the "New Nutrition Science Project" (Cannon and Leitzmann 2006) proposed reframing nutrition and dietetic research and practice around the *interconnected* biological, social and environmental dimensions of nutrition as a science (the term environmental here is used to mean the biological or natural world). The focus on the interconnected dimensions highlighted the need for a "systems approach" to addressing some of nutrition science's more intractable challenges, such as malnutrition, in all its forms. The international support for the New Nutrition Science Project (albeit European Union driven and focused) helped gain attention for the involvement of nutrition in global dialogues on food system sustainability. Ecological nutrition is a term also used to capture such a multidimensional and systems approach now broadly considered necessary to achieving *sustainable diets* (Mason and Lang 2017), which is now gaining policy traction in mainstream dietetics internationally, in Europe (British Dietetic Association 2017), North America (American Dietetic Association 2007; Carlsson et al. 2019); and Australia (Public Health Association Australia 2016). The concept is also emerging more broadly in public health as nations begin to incorporate aspects of sustainability to varying degrees. Qatar, Sweden and Brazil have taken radical steps to embed sustainability and social drivers and determinants into their national dietary guidelines. While dietetic curricula do pay some attention to the food system and sustainable eating, albeit to varying degrees of depth, the dominant focus of dietetic curricula today continues to be on biomedical aspects of nutrition and healthy eating, indicating that dietetic education is unlikely to equip graduates for work in the emerging field of sustainable eating. There is wider consensus that sustainability is an important issue in higher education and a need for all learners to acquire the knowledge and skills needed to promote sustainable development (United Nations General Assembly 2015). Despite this, growing community interest in sustainable eating, and calls for dietitians to bolster food system literacy (Palumbo 2016), barriers remain. Inadequate time in the curriculum (Harmon et al. 2011) and practical training opportunities, including knowledgeable preceptors (Wegener 2018), are two significant barriers to developing competence in this area. Investing in student training and professional development that is grounded in a clear understanding of the terms, concepts and current issues is essential for practitioners to play a strategic role in the future.

Defining Key Terms and Concepts

Sustainable diets (see glossary) is a term that has received increasing attention in the past decade, with roots in these historical eco-dietetic schools of thought and practice; sustainable diets contribute to and are supported by *food system sustainability* (Meybeck and Gitz 2017). The FAO and Bioversity International define sustainable diets as *"… those diets with low environmental impacts which contribute to food and nutrition security and to healthy life for present and future generations. Sustainable diets are protective and respectful of biodiversity and ecosystems, culturally acceptable, accessible, economically fair and affordable; nutritionally adequate, safe and healthy; while optimizing natural and human resources"* (Burlingame and Dernini 2012). The term sustainable diets places emphasis on the notion that human food choices (diets), and in particular those of "Western" and urban consumers, play a pivotal role in *sustainable food systems*.

Sustainable food systems is a broader, though clearly related, term that de-emphasizes the eater while placing more weight on the complex network (sometimes described as a "food chain") of actors that produce, process and distribute food to consumers, often across vast geographic scales. The Food and Agriculture Organization (FAO) defines SFS as those that "…[deliver] food and nutrition security for all in such a way that the economic, social and environmental bases to generate food security and nutrition for future generations are not compromised" (HLPE 2017).

Both definitions are informed by the broadly accepted concept that *sustainability* rests on three main, interconnected systems – (i) the environmental, (ii) social and, in our current reality, (iii) economic. This "systems perspective" helps to see and articulate food systems as a complex network of actors and factors (Norberg and Cumming 2008) interacting with these three domains; it is an important perspective for dietetics because if the implicit values at stake are that we nourish our populations in a way that *does not compromise future generations*, then there is a clear need for dietetic practice to reflect the interrelationship between human diets and the environmental, social and economic impacts of such diets.

While dietetic practice has always put human health as the end goal (and thus the underlying value is that human health is paramount), a true systems perspective requires human health to be balanced against the important needs and limitations of other actors and factors in the system (e.g. other and all people; oceans, soil and air; animals; etc.).

To further challenge dominant dietetic frameworks, one way a systems perspective can be conceptualized is as "nested interdependencies". Fig. 7.1 illustrates the idea that the economy is nested within (dependent on) human society; similarly society is nested within the environment. Food systems are nested within all three systems and here illustrated as a constellation of various-sized actors and factors spanning those three systems.

This nested system perspective is not values-free; it does imply a hierarchy of importance between systems. It begs the question: "do the needs of the environment

Fig. 7.1 A nested systems perspective of food systems

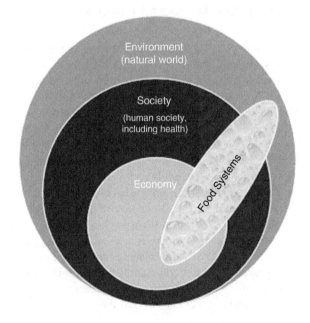

need to be prioritized above social and economic needs?" Further critical thought questions whether, in our current reality of over seven billion people on Earth, environmental integrity is not also dependent on human society being able to meet its own needs. That is to say, as humans we prioritize our needs at the expense of ecological integrity (e.g. we continue to use unsustainably high proportions of the Earth's arable land for human food production at the expense of other needs in the ecosystem). One could argue that, similarly, we assign disproportionate weight and power to the "needs" of the economic system, above those of the social and environmental systems (e.g. governing food systems for profit over equitable access to livelihoods, human health and ecosystems). A systems perspective allows us to see these nested systems (i.e. there is a hierarchy of dependencies) as interdependent (i.e. the systems are interrelated and co-dependent in complex ways).

A Critical Dietetics approach is framed by one that guides practice in a way that is knowledgeable and attentive to the needs and limitations that govern these nested systems.

Unsustainable Nutrition

Food systems are a driving force contributing to ill-health (IPES-Food 2017) and unsustainable conditions in our social and ecological systems.

Food Systems, Ill Health and Inequality

Food systems are contributing to social changes to eating. The food systems in developed countries, and to an increasing extent in developing countries, are largely corporatized and for-profit sitting squarely within capitalist and consumer-oriented societies (Konefal et al. 2005). Citizens are consequently exposed to many highly processed foods that are energy-dense and nutrient poor, which are also priced and marketed to encourage excessive consumption (Lang 2004). Together with social trends towards time pressure and search for quick, easy fixes, these highly processed foods offer convenient, tasty, albeit less healthy, options, which are seen in global dietary trends and concomitant health problems (Jabs and Devine 2006).

Direct relationships between "Western" diets (and the food systems that perpetuate them) and poor health have been well recognized for over 20 years (Drewnowski and Popkin 1997). Western diets are synonymous with diets excessively high in free sugars, salt, fats, meats, and high levels of processing. They are ubiquitous in industrialized nations and, increasingly, in industrializing nations. Transition towards more Western diets is well known to contribute to diet-related diseases, in particular higher risk of type II diabetes, cardiovascular diseases, hypertension (Drewnowski and Popkin 1997) and some cancers (Bouvard et al. 2015).

While over half the world struggles with diet-related, chronic disease, there are inequalities in food access (Lang 2015). We generate more than enough food to feed our current population, just over 7 billion (United Nations 2017), yet approximately 800 million people in the developing world are undernourished, and about 2 billion are deficient in key micronutrients (FAO et al. 2017). Chronic or periodic undernutrition can lead to child stunting or wasting, respectively, which can have intergenerational consequences on the attainment of potential growth and development, with negative social and economic impacts. Deficiency in key micronutrients can lead to acute conditions including blindness and anaemia even in adults. Consequently, the world is facing multiple forms of malnutrition (overnutrition, undernutrition and micronutrient deficiencies) that each carry health burdens. Industrializing countries are struggling with pandemic levels of each, often driven by the nutrition transition, towards Western diets.

Food Systems and Environmental Degradation

A growing human population is increasing demands on our food systems, and at the same time, food systems are stressed by environmental degradation of global ecosystems. But our current food system is also *contributing* to compromised ecosystem resources and services on which our ability to produce food depends (Tilman and Clark 2014). An estimated 20–50% of greenhouse gas emissions (GHGe) are attributed to agricultural activities (Garnett 2011; GRAIN 2011). The bulk of research demonstrates that diets high in red meat (especially from ruminants: cows, sheep, etc.) have a substantial impact on GHGe, even when accounting for variability in production/grazing approaches (Garnett et al. 2017). These GHGe are of central concern to climate change scientists who confirm and predict that climate change is already and will continue to impact our ability to produce food Diets that include higher amounts of animal-sourced foods (commonly meats and dairy products) also use significantly more water (Vanham et al. 2013) and require more land for both pasture and feed (e.g. soy) than would diets with proportionately higher amounts of plant-based foods (e.g. various forms of vegetarian and "flexitarian" diets). With agriculture already using 92% of the global annual average water (Hoekstra and Mekonnen 2012) and land use for human food production at 60% of available land, there is little room to "grow".

These three examples, GHGe, water and land use, provide a meaningful yet incomplete snapshot of the magnitude of food system-related environmental impacts. Taken together with the social and human health-related impacts in the previous section, it becomes clear that implementation of dietary solutions to the tightly linked diet–environment–health trilemma is a challenge on a global scale (Tilman and Clark 2014) requiring a "systems" approach (iPES Food 2015).

With possible co-benefits emerging, more sustainable nutrition lies at the intersection of public health, environmental health and the business of food (Garnett 2014). Food is a massive industry, and the many key players involved have very different interests. There is a call for stronger multi-sector leadership in championing a sustainable ecological approach to food systems (City University of London Centre for Food Policy 2018). Nutrition and dietetic professionals are in a strong position to participate in leading food system sustainability discourse and practice and have a clear role in safeguarding food and nutrition priorities. However, as is discussed in the next section, case examples from the UK, Australia and Canada show that there is a need for a better understanding of their strategic role, and role-specific priorities need to be more strongly articulated. A clearer picture of the professional role will inform training and professional development needs (Pettinger 2018).

For the past number of decades, nutrition and dietetic professionals globally have gained competency working to maximize the diet–health outcomes domain and applying Social Determinants of Health lens to address human health. However, despite the professional history of environmental engagement, addressing ecological determinants of health (e.g. CPHA*ACSP 2015) is mostly considered "out of scope" for health practitioners including dietitians. This is influenced by the dominant neoliberal politics of many countries (including the UK, Australia and Canada), which privilege an individualist focus over a structural (systems) one (Jessop 2016).

To guide nutrition and dietetic education, practice and scholarship, a conceptual framework that guides a transformative curriculum around SFS and diets is needed.

Sustainable Nutrition in Practice

In 2016, the International Congress of Dietetics adopted the theme of 'going to sustainable eating', demonstrating a growing level of interest among dietitians around the globe (and in particular in the European countries, who hosted the Congress). Despite weak and often ad hoc emphasis on the key concepts and issues in education, practice and scholarship in most countries, many dietitians are applying this lens to practice, stepping into non-traditional roles and leadership opportunities to forward this agenda. This section outlines examples from the field in the UK, Australia and Canada, outlining the current situation, (educational) action and outcome for each case presented.

The UK

In the UK, a recently updated sustainable diet policy statement by the British Dietetic Association (BDA) has stated that it believes the profession should be leading discussions on how food behaviours can affect both health *and* the environment (British Dietetic Association 2017). Dietitians, the policy states, are in a strong position to combine healthy eating messages and sustainable dietary advice. This aligns with the newly upgraded UK Eat Well Guide, which mentions sustainability in relation to meat and fish consumption. This BDA policy is accompanied by a practical "toolkit" to support dietitans in practice (BDA, 2018) recently co-created by the BDA with an active group of "special interest" dietitians/nutritionists. Many UK dietitians and nutritionists are already engaged in sustainability advocacy across a range of sectors, for example, working with local food partnerships, a movement that is currently driven by the 'Sustainable Food Cities (place based) Network'. Similarly, some UK dietitians and nutritionists have been involved in sustainability-driven settings-based award schemes, in schools and care home settings, which have seen positive outcomes. Notwithstanding, positive systems-level activity and investment in dietetic student training is important.

Sustainability is being addressed in the dietetic curriculum at the University of Plymouth. An exploratory pedagogic workshop was run with final year dietetic students as part of their Public Health Nutrition module in October 2016 (Pettinger et al. 2018). Student participants ($n = 26$) attended a 2-h workshop, which included: (i) delivery of learning materials by a sustainability specialist dietitian, (ii) basic interactive survey, (iii) group work (discussing potential roles of dietitians in different settings) and (iv) plenary discussion.

The question template was designed based on previous research suggesting a lack of dietetic knowledge about sustainability (Webber and Sarjahani 2011) and supported by responses gathered from a LinkedIn 'straw poll' carried out in spring 2016 asking UK dietitians ($n = 9$) about their broad views on sustainability. This poll indicated above all a lack of definitional clarity around the term 'sustainability' for dietitians. Qualitative feedback was obtained from participating students who demonstrated a reasonable understanding of sustainable eating and could articulate practical roles for dietitians in promoting sustainability, for example, "liaising with [hospital] catering team and minimising food/supplement waste" (student 10). They were enthusiastic to learn about sustainable eating and felt that it should be more strongly embedded in the dietetic curriculum, for example, "it should just be throughout every subject ... so in the 'Dietetics in Practice' module, when we're talking about practical food advice, get us thinking about sustainability, e.g. less meat" (student 5). The views of the students concur with general UK student views (Cotton and Alcock 2013) including that a sustainability lens is needed for curricula that are 'fit for the future'Goodman and East 2014). Interactive participatory workshops align well with adult learning theories for healthcare professionals (Taylor and Hamdy 2013). They have been documented to motivate and energize students, empowering them in transformative learning experiences (Seale 2013). More research is needed to support this educational goal to enable students to be better prepared for the diversity of their future practice. This research is ongoing, currently investigating nutrition/dietetic students' environmental attitudes and how these relate to their actual sustainability practices and behaviours.

Australia

The Dietitians Association of Australia and the Australian Public Health Association (PHAA) have interest groups that engage dietitians and nutritionists on nutrition and sustainability matters. Both groups focus on information sharing, professional development and advocacy. The PHAA has developed explicit policy statements which it uses for advocacy purposes. Public health dietitians advocated for inclusion of sustainable eating into the latest version of the Australian Dietary Guidelines, and, while this is not explicit in the key messages of the guidelines, it nevertheless informed the food modelling and was inserted in the appendices (NHMRC 2013). Notwithstanding professional interest groups, the application of sustainable eating into professional practice by Australian dietitians and nutritionists is largely individualized and voluntary because sustainable eating is not structurally embedded within government food-related policies. At the time of writing this chapter, (2018), Australian governments at all levels have reduced their investment in health promotion and prevention, thereby further marginalizing nutrition sustainability work (Moodie et al. 2016).

Flinders University of South Australia has had a long tradition of critically investigating the food system in its nutrition and dietetic curriculum. It is assumed that this topic is also addressed by other Australian universities. Apart from student education, in 2016, Flinders University academics from Nutrition and Dietetics and Public Health have trialled community education on food systems. They developed a 2-week online course, Food System Matters (FSM), which examined the food system through three lenses: environmental sustainability, fairness and equity and health and nutrition. The curriculum was delivered using a combination of text, videos, images, quizzes, activities, critical thinking questions and discussion forum. The course was delivered through Flinders Learning Online (FLO), Flinders University's internal education platform which limited the trial to staff and students of the university. The education program was evaluated for effects on knowledge about the food system literacy and attitudes to food choices for health (Mehta 2017). Forty-seven staff and students participated in the course and were randomly allocated into one of two groups – (1) Intervention and (2) Control and Intervention. Knowledge about the food system improved significantly for both Intervention groups from baseline ($p < 0.001$) compared to the Control group ($p = 0.00$). Attitudes to sustainable food choices improved significantly for both Intervention groups from baseline ($p < 0.001$; $p = 0.005$) but, however, were not statistically significant when compared to the Control group ($p = 0.065$; $p = 0.43$), although in a positive direction.

Following the quantitative evaluation, a qualitative evaluation was undertaken in 2017, of FSM participants' engagement in sustainable eating behaviours and food system education. Nine tertiary-educated staff participated in the semi-structured interviews. The majority of participants were found to be in the later stages of health behaviour change, in other words, action and maintenance according to the transtheoretical model of behaviour change (Glanz et al. 2015). The FSM course consequently reinforced their existing beliefs and practices about sustainable eating. Participants were primarily motivated by ethics and benefits to broader society which aligns with a US study by Alkon (2008) but contradicts other studies which emphasized values of health, quality, freshness and taste (Hoek et al. 2017). The challenge for community food system literacy is common to all types of health education, namely, to reach those people who are less committed to change by dint of being in the contemplation and pre-contemplation stages of health behaviour change (Hirvonen et al. 2015). Even for the committed participants, time was reported as a barrier to their engagement, and time is known to be a common barrier to participation in health promotion (Linnan et al. 2001).

Food system literacy offers a novel approach to engage the public in a broader discourse on food and society (Lang 2005). Food system literacy has the potential to yield health benefits because food consumption behaviours oriented towards social and environmental sustainability will by default be healthier choices, favouring less meat and processed foods and more locally produced fruits and vegetables (Friel et al. 2014). Notwithstanding the positive outcomes of this pilot community education program, it is not supported by government policy or funding, thereby providing graduates with few opportunities to hone their skills in this subject area.

Canada

In Canada, Dietitians of Canada is beginning to make strategic steps to support Canadian dietitians to be leaders in SFS. In 2015, the Board of Directors of Dietitians of Canada (DC) sets a strategic direction to raise the profile of dietitians as leaders in SFS that promote healthy diets and that involved building a common understanding of what this means, such that dietitians can participate in intersectoral innovations and advocacy. This strategic direction led DC to collaborate on research that began to fulfil these needs and to initiate a SFS Leadership Team to support DC in advocacy and action.

With partners from Acadia University (Canada) and Blekinge Institute for Technology's Department of Strategic Sustainable Development (Sweden), in 2017 DC engaged in research to create common understanding of what we mean when we say "sustainable food systems" and begin to set a course for action. In the research, members of DC were invited to participate in an iterative dialogue through a modified Delphi inquiry process; Carlsson et al. 2019) which asked dietitians to envision a sustainable food system in Canada, describe current barriers and supports, describe high-leverage actions as well as suggest indicators to track progress. This research was in part established to fulfil the needs of the DC SFS Leadership Team, which is currently focused on three key areas: policy and advocacy, education and communication.

The outcomes of the research and the Leadership Team are tied. Of the 4885 DC members invited to participate in the research, over 50 dietitians participated in dialogue over the course of 6 months. Outcomes suggested that high-leverage action areas for dietitians include education, organizational infrastructure/policies and public policy, and key action approaches highlighted the need for reflexive and collaborative approaches (Carlsson et al. 2019). Central to the aim of this chapter was that participating dietitians highlighted the need for education for SFS literacy among dietetic students, professionals and the public. Participating dietitians made it clear that while food systems and sustainability *are* listed as foundational knowledge statement requirements to which all accredited dietetics programs in Canada must adhere (Partnership for Dietetic Education and Practice 2014), dietitians are generally not adequately trained to step into multisectoral innovation for SFS. They identified a need for stronger integration of SFS in dietetic education and training, along with post-graduate professional development opportunities and resources to guide practice, such that dietitians are well equipped to lead the development of programming and policy that will strengthen public SFS literacy.

The need for such education is one of the areas the Leadership Team has chosen to focus on, who, at the time of writing, have developed an evidence review on plant-based diets and the environment, which will form the basis of future practice resources, and discussions at national conference on setting strategic directions, speaking about sustainability in language accessible to the audience, plant-based diets in institutions and the role of dietitians in sustainable diets. The Leadership Team has also been actively advocating for national food policy that applies a systems lens, for example, through explicit messages about sustainability in national food guidance.

While there is still much work to be done, the member-informed and member-led approach that Dietitians of Canada is taking shows promise for increasing interest in SFS as a practice area and competence to lead innovations for food system sustainability.

These three case study examples illustrate movement (in the right direction) globally in this essential field for dietitians. Yet all three highlight obvious educational gaps that need to be urgently filled, if the future dietetic workforce is going to be adequately equipped with the skills required to contribute to SFS.

Moving Forward

What Is the Role for Dietitians?

Dietitians have an important role in advising the public around sustainable diets as well as addressing the many challenges of building a more resilient and sustainable food system. In the US, this role is recognized and defined by the publication of the professional position paper 'Standards for Professional Performance for Registered Dietitian Nutritionist in Sustainable, Resilient, and Healthy Food and Water Systems' (Tagtow 2014).

Given some of the evidence reviewed under the section on Unsustainable Nutrition, linking food systems to human health, food culture and environmental degradation and given the globally interdependent nature of these complex issues, the role of nutrition professionals is more significant and pressing than ever, and international coordination is advisable. But for this to happen, there needs to be an agreement from international and national dietetic/nutrition professional bodies that sustainability/food system literacy is an essential part of education, training and practice.

The case examples in this chapter illustrate that there are several key leverage points where nutrition and dietetic professionals can make meaningful, systematic change: (1) advocacy and public policy, (2) influencing organizational policies and structures and (3) education and training for both nutrition professionals as well as the public. In this section we discuss the third leverage point – education and training – and explore emerging barriers and supports. Given the reciprocal relationship of influence between curricula in accredited dietetics programs and evidence-based professional practice, the below discussion mingles the opportunities and challenges for dietetic students and professionals alike.

The Need for Education and Training

There are international and national-level calls for general sustainability education to meet the United Nations Sustainable Development Goals, as well as specific calls related to health professionals. Currently dietetic education and training does not equip present and future professionals for leadership roles in SFS and diets (Pettinger). Harmon et al. (2011) has highlighted the need to develop foundational educational knowledge and skill competencies for nutrition professionals related to food systems and sustainability, and it has been described as an obligatory professional growth area by Wegener (2018).

There is emerging evidence that integration of even short-term sustainability education into formal education can be an effective tool for public education, as illustrated by the Australian case example, as well as dietetic trainees. Innes et al. (2018) looked at the integration of 'environmental literacy' in undergraduate nutrition programs in the USA and found that a 2-week food sustainability module improved student sustainable literacy levels. These two examples support the utility of formalized sustainability education, in particular in concentrated modules that may be easier and faster to implement than holistic curriculum changes, and an opportunity for dietetic education and training, as well as continued professional development models.

However, a Critical Dietetics approach would challenge dietetic educators to apply a more systematic approach – using a 'sustainability lens' through which to view the development of nutrition and dietetic education, practice and scholarship that are:

- Grounded in a clear understanding of the terms, concepts and current issues
- Knowledgeable and attentive to the needs, limitations and interdependencies of the economic, social and environmental systems
- Guided by a conceptual framework that facilitates critical analysis of complex systems approaches

The Approach

A Critical Dietetics approach would also be reflexive – moving forward with new ways of thinking about evidence – and collaborative, with expanded notions of what other expertise is relevant to our work.

New ways of thinking about evidence are necessary. There are some nutrition professionals already championing leadership in this area, who recognize the paradigm shift that accompanies the advancing wave of complexity thinking which emphasizes 'non-linear' contexts and promotes 'systems thinking' approaches to problem-solving. There is a fundamental challenge, however, for nutrition/dietetic education, which has its traditions in biomedical models of evidence-based practice relying on mainly reductionist research paradigms. Extending the remit of evidence-based practice to embrace more relational models of critical thinking is needed in all nutrition training and practice. The Critical Dietetics movement "seeks to explore new ways of framing how we educate, practice and research in dietetics, i.e., the professional discipline of nutrition" (Gingras et al. 2014). This postulates the need to expand traditional theoretical frameworks beyond current conventional thinking. Nutrition professionals, therefore, should be bringing critical perspectives on food and health (in their broadest sense) to sustainability.

Dietitians are accustomed to collaborating in multidisciplinary teams (e.g. other health professionals, community services, urban planning, etc.). In the area of food systems sustainability, collaborations with less familiar sectors can present new challenges and opportunities, perhaps even conflicts of interest, if, for example, work is being carried out with the private sector (Johnston and Finegood 2015). Regardless, an openness to knowledge, evidence and experience together with non-traditional knowledge domains and colleagues is important to meaningful learning and progress. We cannot be experts in all the relevant socioecological domains; but by learning to learn from and collaborate with others, practitioners and members of the public may approach a more reflexive, systems approach.

What Are the Barriers?

While arguing for systematic integration of a critical sustainability lens in dietetic education, and practice, we recognize that there are known barriers, which need to be acknowledged. These can be categorized as sociopolitical, professional and institutional.

Sociopolitical Barriers

The governments of Australia, the UK and Canada can be described as neo-liberal, to the extent that economics is at the heart of the conduct of government; free markets are perceived to be essential to the success of the sovereign state and its population (Dean 2010). Neo-liberalism maintains the governance role of the state at a level which is moderate, frugal and prudent. Not unexpectedly, in neo-liberal societies, the food industry exerts considerable influence on matters of governance (such as national dietary guidance), upholding its profit-making interests even when this conflicts with public interest. Citizens in neo-liberal societies are considered to be autonomous individuals, with the freedom to choose; however, these rights come with responsibilities for self-regulation, e.g. to make food choices that contribute to wellbeing (Bauman, 2009). Dietitians, as the experts using disciplinary knowledge and technologies, reinforce food industry-informed, publicly encouraged (through, e.g., dietary guidance) behaviours through education, monitoring and surveillance of citizens. In this way, dietetics has adapted uncritically to the dominant individualistic discourse and evolved to work with the autonomous, self-regulating individual, rather than problematizing structures or systems. Further, this societal discourse presents a challenge as the public too is embedded in this discourse (Mehta 2013).

Professional Barriers

While there is evidence of growing interest and engagement, there are mixed levels of competence. Some researchers have found that there appears to be a reasonable understanding of the broad conceptual definitions of sustainable eating, while others indicate a lack of knowledge, practical skills and competence to work confidently on SFS. Predictably, a small sample of student dietitians reported that they do not have the confidence in their knowledge to apply it effectively (Pettinger et al. 2018), even though they wanted to engage with the topic.

This is exacerbated by the lack of clarity on the complex terms and concepts and reinforced by apparent conflicting perspectives about communicating information on sustainable diets and eating. Consumers are influenced by nutrition and health messages from a range of different sources, some of them with conflicts of interest, for example, between profit and consumer wellbeing and social or environmental outcomes. The sustainable diet agenda is likely to add to the plethora of messaging, and potentially confuse consumers further (Mason and Lang 2017), and thus an opportunity for dietitians, who are skilled in effective public education, to engage.

Furthermore, in the UK, the relevance of SFS and diets is not uniformly clear across different population groups (e.g. vulnerable groups) yet alone in the various dietetic practice settings and concern that these priorities might conflict with nutrition therapy priorities. Perceived lack of relevance and cultural authority to act will be a barrier to meaningful integration of a SFS lens in how dietitians work with interns, colleagues (including those from other disciplines) and the public to frame problems.

Institutional Barriers

In most countries that offer accredited programs in universities, dietetic curricula are driven by professional standards. This offers significant advantages in terms of the credibility of the profession. But as discussed previously, one fundamental challenge is that these professional standards are shaped by scientific evidence rooted in biomedical models of evidence analysis, as well as neoliberal governance models, which don't lend themselves well to complex socioecological challenges such as unsustainable nutrition.

Furthermore, practical issues such as time and space in the curriculum are perceived as significant barriers to expanding teaching on food systems and sustainability. Despite universal acknowledgement that a wide range of skills and knowledge are required to create an action-orientated sustainability-literate graduate body, many of these skills and attributes are inadequately addressed in dietetic curricula because the already tight curricula prioritize competency specifications of professional dietetic bodies.

Conclusion

While the barriers are many, the case examples in this chapter highlight examples of sustainability education being incorporated into dietetic and public education as well as practice. These demonstrate the potential of emerging examples of the application of a sustainability lens in dietetic education, the use of formal education approaches, settings-based motivational programs for public education on food systems sustainability as well as efforts on the part of professional dietetic associations working to embed these issues into the organizational culture. To build on these, and other successes, there is a need for a Critical Dietetics approach: one that is based on values where individual health, the health of the society (social system) and ecosystem health are of equal importance; one that moves beyond the biosciences to a conceptual framework that guides transdisciplinary and transformative education for nutrition students, practitioners and the public.

Assignments

Level 1: Understanding key concepts.
Compile your own glossary of terms based on any concepts that are unfamiliar to
   you (try to make them evidence based where possible).

Level 2: Reflect on and apply key concepts in a new context.
Reflect on your experience as a nutrition and dietetics student thus far. In what ways
   could a Critical Dietetics approach to SFS and diets have been integrated into
   some of your learning opportunities (course work, practical training, etc.)?
Imagine yourself practising within the following dietetic/nutrition settings. Describe
   opportunities to apply sustainable diet/food system thinking to your role: E.g. of
   roles (public health, industry, community, clinical, media or other role that is
   emerging or relevant in your home country)?

Level 3: Analyse and critique the concepts.
Moving beyond the focus on educational aspects, write a critical analysis of the
   nutrition professional/dietitian roles in (1) advocacy and public policy and (2)
   influencing organizational policies and structures.

Definition of Keywords and Terms

Ecological nutrition   A term used to capture such a multidimensional and
                              systems approach now broadly considered necessary to
                              achieving *sustainable diets*.
Sustainable diets   The FAO and Bioversity International define sustain-
                              able diets as *"… those diets with low environmental
                              impacts which contribute to food and nutrition security
                              and to healthy life for present and future generations.
                              Sustainable diets are protective and respectful of biodi-
                              versity and ecosystems, culturally acceptable, accessi-
                              ble, economically fair and affordable; nutritionally
                              adequate, safe and healthy; while optimizing natural
                              and human resources"*.
Sustainable food systems   The Food and Agriculture Organization (FAO) defines
                              SFS as those that "…[deliver] food and nutrition secu-
                              rity for all in such a way that the economic, social and
                              environmental bases to generate food security and
                              nutrition for future generations are not compromised"
                              (HLPE 2017).

References

Alkon AH (2008) From value to values: sustainable consumption at farmers markets. Agric Hum Values 25:487–498. https://doi.org/10.1007/s10460-008-9136-

Bauman Z (2009) Does Ethics Have a Chance in a World of Consumers. Harvard University Press, Cambridge, UK

Beauman C, Cannon G, Elmadfa I et al The principles, definition and dimensions of the new nutrition science. Public Health Nutr 8:695–698

Bouvard V, Loomis D, Guyton KZ et al (2015) Carcinogenicity of consumption of red and processed meat. Lancet Oncol 16:1599–1600. https://doi.org/10.1016/S1470-2045(15)00444-1

British Dietetic Association (2017) British Dietetic Association Policy Statement: Sustainable Diets

British Dietetic Association (2018) One Blue Dot: Environmentally Sustainable Diet Toolkit/Reference guide for dietitians https://www.bda.uk.com/professional/resources/environmentally_sustainable_diet_toolkit_-_one_blue_dot

Burlingame B, Dernini S (2012) Sustainable diets and biodiversity: directions and solutions for policy, research and action. Nutrition and consumer protection division, food and agriculture organization, Rome, Italy

Cannon G, Leitzmann C (2006) The new nutrition science project. Scand J Food Nutr 50:5–12

Carlsson L, Callaghan E, Broman G (2019) How can dietitians leverage change for sustainable foodsystems in Canada? Can J Diet Pract Res.

City University of London Centre for Food Policy (2018) Food Research Collaboration. http://foodresearch.org.uk/about-us/. Accessed 31 Jul 2018

Cotton DR, Alcock I (2013) Commitment to environmental sustainability in the UK student population. Stud High Educ 38:1457–1471. https://doi.org/10.1080/03075079.2011.627423

CPHA*ACSP (2015) Global change and public health: addressing the ecological determinants of health. Canadian Public Health Association, Ottawa, ON

Dean M (2010) Governmentality: power and rule in mondern society, 2nd edn. Sage Publications, London

Drewnowski A, Popkin BM (1997) The nutrition transition: new trends in the global diet. Nutr Rev 55:31–43

Dyball R, Carlsson L (2017) Ellen Swallow Richards: mother of human ecology? Hum Ecol Rev 23:17–28

FAO, IFAD, UNICEF, et al. (2017) The State of Food Security and Nutrition in the World, 2017. Building resilience for peace and food security. Food and Agriculture Organization of the United Nations, Rome, FAO

Friel S, Barosh LJ, Lawrence M (2014) Towards healthy and sustainable food consumption: an Australian case study. Public Health Nutr 17:1156–1166. https://doi.org/10.1017/S1368980013001523

Garnett T (2011) Where are the best opportunities for reducing greenhouse gas emissions in the food system (including the food chain)? Food Policy 36:S23–S32. https://doi.org/10.1016/j.foodpol.2010.10.010

Garnett T (2014) Three perspectives on sustainable food security: efficiency, demand restraint, food system transformation. What role for life cycle assessment? J Clean Prod 73:10–18. https://doi.org/10.1016/j.jclepro.2013.07.045

Garnett T, Godde C, Muller A, et al. (2017) Grazed and confused. Food climate research network

Gingras J, Asada Y, Fox A et al (2014) Critical Dietetics: a discussion paper, vol 2, pp 2–12

Glanz K, Rimer BK, Viswanath K (2015) Health behavior: theory, research, and practice, 5th edn. Jossey-Bass, San Francisco, CA

Goodman B, East L (2014) The "sustainability lens": a framework for nurse education that is "fit for the future". Nurse Educ Today 34:100–103 doi: 0.1016/j.nedt.2013.02.010

GRAIN (2011) Food and climate change: the forgotten link. https://www.grain.org/article/entries/4357-food-and-climate-change-the-forgotten-link. Accessed 16 Jun 2016

Gussow JD, Clancy KL (1986) Dietary guidelines for sustainability. J Nutr Educ 18:1–5

Harmon A, Lapp JL, Blair D, Hauck-Lawson A (2011) Teaching food system sustainability in dietetic programs: need, conceptualization, and practical approaches. J Hunger Environ Nutr 6:114–124

Hirvonen N, Korpelainen R, Pyky R, Huotari M-L (2015) Health information literacy and stage of change in relation to physical activity information seeking and avoidance: a population-based study among young men. In: Proceedings of the 78th ASIS&T Annual Meeting. American Society for Information Science, Silver Springs, MD, USA

HLPE (2017) Nutrition and Food Systems. A report by the High Level Panel of Experts on Food Security and Nutrition of the Committee on World Food Security. Committee on World Food Security, Rome

Hoek A, Pearson D, James S et al (2017) Shrinking the food-print: a qualitative study into consumer perceptions, experiences and attitudes towards healthy and environmentally friendly food behaviours. Appetite 2017:117–131. https://doi.org/10.1016/j.appet.2016.09.030

Hoekstra AY, Mekonnen MM (2012) The water footprint of humanity. Proc Natl Acad Sci 109:3232. https://doi.org/10.1073/pnas.1109936109

Innes S, Shephard K, Furnari M et al (2018) Greening the curriculum to foster environmental literacy in tertiary students studying human nutrition. J Hunger Environ Nutr 13:192–204. https://doi.org/10.1080/19320248.2016.1255693

iPES Food (2015) The new science of sustainable food systems: overcoming barriers to food systems reform

IPES-Food (2017) Unravelling the Food-Health Nexus: addressing practices, political economy, and power relations to build healthier food systems. The Global Alliance for the Future of Food and IPES-Food

Jabs J, Devine C (2006) Time scarcity and food choices: an overview. Appetite 47:196–204

Jessop RD (2016) The handbook of neoliberalism: the heartlands of neoliberalism and the rise of the Austerity State, S Springer, K Birch & L McLeavy. Routledge

Johnston L, Finegood D (2015) Cross-sector partnerships and public health: challenges and opportunities for adressing obesity and noncommunicable diseases through engagement with the private sector. Annu Rev Public Health 18:255–271. https://doi.org/10.1146/annurev-publhealth-031914-122802

Konefal J, Mascarenhas M, Hatanaka M (2005) Governance in the global agro-food system: backlighting the role of transnational supermarket chains. Agric Hum Values 22:291–302

Lang T (2004) Food industrialisation and food power: implications for food governance. Dev Policy Rev 21:555–568. https://doi.org/10.1111/j.1467-8659.2003.00223.x

Lang T (2005) Food control or food democracy? Re-engaging nutrition with society and the environment. Public Health Nutr 8:730–737

Lang T (2015) In: Earthscan, from Routledge (ed) Food wars: the global battle for mouths, minds and markets, 2nd edn, London\New York

Linnan L, Sorensen G, Colditz G et al (2001) Using theory to understand the multiple determinants of low participation in worksite health promotion programs. Health Educ Behav 28:591–607

Mason P, Lang T (2017) Sustainable diets: how ecological nutrition can transform consumption and the food system. Routledge, New York

Mehta K (2013) Parents' and children's perceptions of food and beverage marketing to which children are exposed. Flinders University

Meybeck A, Gitz V (2017) Sustainable diets within sustainable food systems. Proc Nutr Soc 76:1–11. https://doi.org/10.1017/S0029665116000653

Moodie AR, Tolhurst P, Martin JE (2016) Australia's health: being accountable for prevention. Med J Aust 205:223–225. https://doi.org/10.5694/mja15.00968

NHMRC (2013) Australian dietary guidelines. National Health and Medical Research Council, Canberra

Norberg J, Cumming GS (2008) Complexity theory for a sustainable future. Columbia University Press, New York

Palumbo R (2016) Sustainability of well-being through literacy. The effects of food literacy on sustainability of well-being. Agric Agric Sci Procedia 8:99–106. https://doi.org/10.1016/j.aaspro.2016.02.013

Partnership for Dietetic Education and Practice (2014) Standards - PDEP. https://www.pdep.ca/tools/standards.aspx. Accessed 13 Jun 2018

Pettinger C (2018) Sustainable eating: opportunities for nutrition professionals. Nutrition Bulletin

Pettinger C, Atherton E, Miller W (2018) Engaging student dietitians in 'sustainability principles' throughout the curriculum: an exploratory pedagogic workshop. J Nutr Diet 31:44

Position of the American Dietetic Association (2007) Food and Nutrition Professionals Can Implement Practices to Conserve Natural Resources and Support Ecological Sustainability. Journal of the American Dietetic Association 107 (6):1033-1043Mehta K (2017) Promoting community awareness of the food system: benefits and risks. Dietit Assoc Aust SA Branch, Professioanl development workshop

Public Health Association Australia (2016) Public Health Association of Australia: Policy-at-a-glance – Ecologically Sustainable Population for Australia Policy

Rebrovick T (2015) The politics of diet: "eco-dietetics," neoliberalism, and the history of dietetic discourses. Polit Res Q Salt Lake City 68:678–689

Seale J (2013) Doing student voice work in higher education: an exploration of the value of participatory methods. Br Educ Res J 36:995–1015. https://doi.org/10.1080/01411920903342038

Tagtow A (2014) Academy of Nutrition and Dietetics: Standards of professional performance for Registered Dietitian Nutritionists (Competent, Proficient, and Expert) in Sustainable, Resilient, and Healthy Food and Water Systems. J Acad Nutr Diet 114:475–488.e24

Taylor D, Hamdy H (2013) Adult learning theories: implications for learning and teaching in medical education: AMEE Guide NO 83. Med Teach 35:1561–1572. https://doi.org/10.3109/0142159X.2013.828153

Tilman D, Clark M (2014) Global diets link environmental sustainability and human health. Nature 515:518–522. https://doi.org/10.1038/nature13959

United Nations (2017) World Population Prospects: The 2017 Revision | Multimedia Library – United Nations Department of Economic and Social Affairs. In: UN Dep Econ Soc Aff. https://www.un.org/development/desa/publications/world-population-prospects-the-2017-revision.html. Accessed 13 Jun 2018

United Nations General Assembly (2015) Transforming our world: the 2030 Agenda for Sustainable Development

Vanham D, Mekonnen MM, Hoekstra AY (2013) The water footprint of the EU for different diets. Ecol Indic 32:1–8. https://doi.org/10.1016/j.ecolind.2013.02.020

Webber CB, Sarjahani A (2011) Fitting sustainable food systems into dietetic internships—a growing trend. J Hunger Environ Nutr 6:477–489. https://doi.org/10.1080/19320248.2011.627304

Wegener J (2018) Equipping future generations of registered dietitian nutritionists and public health nutritionists: a commentary on education and training needs to promote sustainable food systems and practices in the 21st century. J Acad Nutr Diet 118:393. https://doi.org/10.1016/j.jand.2017.10.024

Suggested Readings

Food Climate Research Network's *Foodsource*: Evidence-based resources on SFS. Foodsource's purpose is to build the foundations for this understanding and for change towards more SFS, by increasing food systems literacy

Mason P, Lang T (2017b) Sustainable diets: how ecological nutrition can transform cosumption and the food system. Earthscan, Abingdon

Chapter 8
'Eating Right': Critical Dietetics, Dietitians and Ethics

John Coveney

Aim of Chapter and Learning Outcomes

The aim of this chapter is:

- To explore various understandings of ethical principles for dietetic practice
- To examine the ways that critical dietetics applies ethics to core values in dietetic practice

At the end of this chapter, readers will:

(i) Describe the ethical principles that guide critical dietetics.
(ii) Apply different understandings of ethics to clinical and community dietetic practice.
(iii) Appreciate the implications of applying the principles of critical dietetics to ethical situations.

Summary

Ethical issues are usually brought to dietetic practices through ethical principles that are supported by professional associations. The purpose of ethics is to encourage best practice and respectful relationships between professionals and their various patients and communities. A broader understanding of ethics situates practices within particular forms of knowledge and within particular cultures. What may pass as ethical and eating 'right' in one situation may not be so clear in another. An appreciation of the fundamental concepts in dietetic practices and the assumptions

J. Coveney (✉)
Flinders University, Adelaide, SA, Australia
e-mail: john.coveney@flinders.edu.au

© Springer Nature Switzerland AG 2019
J. Coveney, S. Booth (eds.), *Critical Dietetics and Critical Nutrition Studies*,
Food Policy, https://doi.org/10.1007/978-3-030-03113-8_8

that are embedded within these practices provides an opportunity to explore ways of appreciating critical dietetics principles.

Introduction

We met as planned at Lunel station. I thought the train would be late and would upset our plans to shop at Les Halles in Lunel central. But no, it arrived right on time. Louis was standing at the platform, looking for my familiar face. It was good to see him there. We greeted each other in the familiar southern France manner and headed over to his car. As we climbed in, we offered each other the usual salutations about how well are you doing and how is life right now. For Louis this is always a tricky question. He is an architect, and his life is influenced by his work, which comes in peaks and troughs. So his response is often unexpected, when he tells you how good (plentiful) or not good (bleak) is his work load.

Sunday morning in Lunel central is wonderful, always very crowded, with the pavement cafes full of folk sunning themselves in the morning sunshine. But being crowded brings its own problems, especially with parking and finding somewhere to put the car. Louis' familiarity with Lunel meant that he fell back on experience which gave him the chance to find something others would not have noticed. Lunel is probably typical of small to medium towns in southern France. A main square with lots of cafes, shops, official buildings taking up most of the space.

Out of the car and into the food hall. Bags in hand. First stop the poissonnerie (fish stall) for ingredients of an entrée we would be eating at lunch. Oyster, prawns, periwinkles. I watch Louis' trained eye move slowly over the offerings. I saw his nose twitch as he sniffed the air that told him how long the shell fish had been out of water. His eyes moved onto an adjacent stall selling much the same products and, to my untrained eye, what looked to be very similar degrees of freshness. But Louis obviously saw differently. A look of satisfaction told me he was more satisfied with offerings over here. Similar experience at the fruit and vegetable stalls. He seems to know what is available and where. He also seems to know what is in season and thus what is to be bought and thus cooked. At an earlier visit, I expressed an interest in cardoons, which I had never eaten. Louis told me this was the cardoon season, so I toured the local fruit and vegetable shops arriving eventually at one with reliable supply which then comprised the central dish that evening. I offered to buy the cheese. What would be reliable and suitable for our meal which we would cook and eat together later? The aged Cantal would be good and some soft goat cheese. That will do just fine. Back to the car with bags heaving. Homeward bound.

What was obvious here was the sense of experience, trust in decisions and engagement directly with the food that we were buying. Louis seemed to bring all his senses to the experience of deciding what to eat and choosing the best ingredients. Because most of the food came unprocessed even unwrapped, there were no signatures or signposts on labels that could be used to guide choice or purchase. What mattered here was the direct engagement with the food and bringing to that the years of observation, experience and with this a confidence in food purchasing. But not only in the buying of food because in the kitchen later, the same levels of experience and know-how were also on show.

The dominance of the central fridges, cold cabinets and the racks and shelves of packaged food products – and a strange yet familiar odour – was the hallmark of the shopping experience with Katy. We agreed to meet at the entrance to a large shopping mall and go off to the supermarket together. Katy was fitting our meeting into her busy architect practice schedule and was shopping for a family of four, including two children under 10 years old and one of them – the 4-year-old – in a tow. Katy made it clear that food shopping was not her favourite activity, especially with an accompanying child. So there was a need to be efficient and well-organised. But, hey, no cutting corners and going for the quick and dirties because like most parents and food providers, Katy wanted to ensure that family meals were healthy and tasty. After cruising through the fruit and vegetable section, near the entrance, like almost all supermarkets, we find ourselves at the fridges. Katy finds that the shelves with her usual brands of yoghurt and cheese are empty. So she is in the process of finding others. Her eyes scanning the alternative offerings, Katy finds herself choosing between one product over another. The labels of each are replete with information about contents and provenance. But the most important decision maker is the Health Star Rating[1] that occupies almost a third of the front of pack. No need to dwell on the decision for too long because the one with 4 stars is a clear winner over the others, 3 stars and 3.5 stars, respectively. Katy finds herself applying this logic, based on science, to almost all her food purchasing decisions. That is to say, she relies on a scientific appraisal of the food, relayed through the Health Star Rating system, to inform her about the quality of the food she is purchasing. 'Quality' here means nutritional contents.

We are out of the supermarket in super quick time and back to her car where we load up the boot with our bought items.

Different Appraisals of Eating 'Right'

So, we have descriptions here of two shopping expeditions separated by geographical distance, culture and language. But the main separation is between an appraisal of food quality relying on experience, familiarity and know-how or rather different types of experience, familiarity and know-how. For Louis, his repository of knowledge about food, accumulated over years of shouldering the family responsibility for food provisioning, is employed to seek out and choose what he understood to be

---

[1] Health Star Rating systems are common in many jurisdictions. In Australia and New Zealand, Health Star Ratings provide a front of pack label that summarises the nutritional quality of the food. Ratings range from ½ star to 5 stars depending on the content of macronutrients and energy. For a full description of Health Star Ratings in Australia and New Zealand, see: http://healthstar-rating.gov.au/internet/healthstarrating/publishing.nsf/Content/About-health-stars.

quality. His knowingness of and familiarity with the offerings at Les Halles allowed him to be in command of his food purchases. For Katy, there is another kind of knowingness, one informed by nutritional science, and ipso facto, requiring deciphering to make it intelligible for the majority of shoppers. Katy needed to have the nutrition facts and figures concentrated into one visual representation: the Health Star Rating system. But there is another difference between the two shopping experiences. Louis' culture, that of the French food culture, will have supplied him with the products of centuries of *savoir* and *connaissance*: know-how and know what. The Cantal cheese, the goat cheese and many of the other purchases come from a long historical line of food production and food manufacturing. Granted some of these may have been modernised and industrialised, even so one can see elements of an unchanging process, like the chestnut leaves that are wrapping the goat cheese, a practice that harks back to the time when these cheeses were wrapped and stored over winter months. That is to say, Louis lives in a deep food culture. Deep in terms of its history and its tradition.

Coming from a 'soft' food culture, Katy relies on very different senses and sensibilities. With no roots to anchor her food practices into history and tradition, Katy uses modern methods of knowledge – based on scientific more modern rationalities – to inform her decision-making processes. In this way she is reliant less on her own innate experiences and expertise and more on the scientific knowledge embedded in and displayed by the Health Star Rating system. She is, by this fact, a more passive shopper.

Critical Dietetics, Dietitians and Ethics

Normally dietitians deal with ethics in terms of professional practice. That is to say, they abide by rules of practice and codes of conduct that require them to perform in particular ways. Accordingly, the ethics of practising dietitians in Australia are governed by the national professional association, the Dietitians Association of Australia. Like professional associations in other jurisdictions, DAA requires members to perform practices that are legal, safe, accountable, honest, fair, non-exploitative and non-discriminatory and promote ecological, social and economic environments that support health and wellbeing. However, ethics has another more culturally bound meaning which is concerned with the individual's disposition to 'do the right thing'. In this case, the right thing is whatever is taken to be the correct moral attitude or form of moral action. The shopping expeditions of Louis and of Katy comprise different understandings of what is 'right to eat'. This is not to assume that in France there is no scientific understanding of food as 'nutrition' and that knowledge of this does not guide food shopping or eating or to assume that in Katy's home state in Australia, there is no place that promotes more gastronomic food provisions.

However, we need to recognise that the 'norms' in either jurisdiction dictate what the ethical – or proper – modes of behaviour. Clearly dietetics and dietitians in each jurisdiction, France and Australia, need to recognise that the rules of engagement with food and with eaters will be different or rather appropriate to each culture. There are, however, some overarching principles that transcend culture, and these are explained below.

Dietetics has been an expanding field of professional practice, research, education and training in Australia and overseas. With roots in the nineteenth-century home economics movement, and in large-scale catering for medical, military and other institutional purposes, dietetics today engages with clinical, community and industry aspects of practice. Although it has obvious links to nutrition, dietetics distinguishes itself through a particular focus on the therapeutic relationship between nutrients, health and disease in humans. That is to say, dietetics is not merely interested in understanding the role of food components in metabolic and physiological systems but specifically in the ways in which health can be optimised, disease can be minimised and illness can be rectified through diet. The interest in food and in the body provides dietetics with potential scope of engagement that goes beyond studying nutrients and their metabolic fate. And because dietitians engage with people and their 'bodies', they have ethical responsibilities to ensure that they practice legal, safe, honest, non-discriminatory methods in dealing with patients, clients, communities, etc.

However, 'food', 'health' and 'bodies' are problematic concepts in the sense that there is not, cannot, and should not be one singular understanding of them as either individual entities or as entities in interaction. The emergence of obesity as an 'epidemic' provides a good example of the ways in which broader interests in food and the body have entered into the debates on overweight. It would be fair to say that, until recently, research and scholarship into overweight have been confined to disciplines in the biosciences like medicine and dietetics and to some social sciences, especially psychology. Now, scholarly contributions to the issue are just as likely to come from broader social sciences, humanities and even science and engineering, as from the traditional host discipline of bioscience. This example demonstrates that potential interest in the relationships between food and the body extends across academia.

Critical dietetics is broadly interested in, but not limited to, four core questions:

- What are the relationships between food and the body that nourish physical, mental, moral/ethical and spiritual existence?
- From where do these relationships derive?
- What are the appropriate ways of studying these relationships?
- What are the appropriate ways towards teaching and learning about these relationships for professional practice?

The first question, *What are the relationships between food and the body that nourish physical, mental, moral/ethical and spiritual existence?*, is one of ontology. Critical dietetics seeks to understand the existence of multiple roles and functions that food plays in individual and social experiences. This understanding cannot be divorced from the body as a 'thing' in culture. So the interconnectedness of food and bodies is of paramount importance to critical dietetics. The ethical questions here derive from the acknowledgement that dietitians will need to deal with patients, clients and communities with specific ontological assumptions that may not accord with the findings or dictates of modern nutritional science which underpins conventional dietetic practice. Going to our two shopping expeditions presented earlier, how might 'eating right' and advice about that be tailored to the needs of Louis and of Katy? Or is there a 'one size fits all'?

The second question, *From where do these relationships derive?*, is one of epistemology. The definition of epistemology concerns bodies of knowledge that render certain phenomena as knowable and are culturally and historically constructed. Critical dietetics explores the genealogy of knowledges concerning food, the body, health and disease and the conditions under which these knowledges gain legitimacy and power. This requires a study of the institutionalisation, training and practice of dietetics and the actors who take part. Critical dietetics may call into question the ways in which the food supply supports a plethora of industries, some private and some public, the necessary resources that keep those industries running and the knowledges that underpin them.

In the case of the two shopping expeditions described earlier, it may be said that for Louis, he is selecting from a short food chain. That is to say, the products that he is choosing are mostly locally grown, locally manufactured and locally sold. Thus, the path from producer to consumer is relatively limited in length by virtue of food traditions and history in which eating locally has been a virtue of French culture. For Katy, the food chain is arguably longer. The food system from which she selects food is one where the distance between producers and consumers has grown longer and more complex. As we can see from the methods employed by Louis and Katy, respectively, to know food and make food choices, they rely on different knowledges, one observational and empirical and the other scientistic and technological. Thus, the ethical question is: which one would dietitians support and how would they come to that decision?

It is probably the case that food systems in Katy's world did, traditionally, look much like the food world of Louis, described above. Yet, with the modernisation of lifestyles, the increasing importance of work outside the home and the prioritisation of urgencies that require time and attention away from food and eating, we see a change in the ways in which food is selected, appraised and purchased. This move from a more holistic, gastronomic approach of food selection based on tradition and empiricism (taken here to mean experience) to one more industrialised and technically rational could be described as 'disenchantment'. Briefly, this is a term coined mostly by sociologist Max Weber to describe the move from a religious to a more secular foundation of society. But the term has been used by other scholars who want to examine how social relationships have moved from a foundation of traditions, faith and customs to ones which are informed by scientific principles and rationalities. For example, in her book *The Disenchantment of the Home*, Kerreen Reiger shows how, in Australia, scientific and calculated ways of managing the domestic space and households – rearing children, caring for home, food provisioning, etc. – took hold during the years between World War I and World War II. The resulting technical rationality rewrote the tasks of parents – especially women and mothers. We can see similar developments in the area of food and nutrition, where one's experience of food and cooking in ways that were traditional and even time honoured has given way to practices that are more informed by science and technology.

The third question, *What are the appropriate ways of studying these relationships?*, is one of methodology. Critical dietetics is as interested in the justification for methods of enquiry as in the findings from such endeavours. One crucial aspect of methodology here is reflexivity. This has to be the case given that critical dietetics is not wedded to one particular theoretical approach but is rather pre-paradigmic. Thus, a concerted effort to understand the role of the researcher and practitioner in formulating questions and seeking answers is crucial to critical dietetics. Further to this is understanding how we approach and appraise the different ways of knowing. For example, coming to the two shopping scenarios painted earlier, Katy's world of knowing food and understanding its relationship to health and wellbeing would be informed by the logic, rationale and techniques of nutrition and technology. Using these instruments of knowledge, it would be possible to understand the ingredients of food by virtue of macro- and micronutrient content, whereas, for Louis it is likely that his gastronomic knowledge and, importantly, experience would be applied to the appreciation of flavour, texture, gastronomic compatibility and seasonal suitability. These are characteristics that are difficult to calibrate. So the ethical issue for dietitians is which source of knowledge to privilege.

The fourth question, *What are the appropriate ways towards teaching and learning about these relationships for professional practice?*, is one of pedagogy. Critical dietetics is committed to extending current content in and processes of professional training. Students and teachers become co-learners and co-teachers in understanding the complexities of the physical, biological and social world in which practice takes place. Such a pedagogy reinforces the experience in professional practice, where practitioners and their patients or their communities take part in a respectful process of sharing knowledge, experience and aspirations leading to better nutritional and emotional health and wellbeing for all. But co-learning brings with it a number of ethical questions, one of which is the issue of power. Professional training and education invariable comes with hierarchies of status, and although the power implications of these hierarchies can be ameliorated to some extent, they can never be fully extinguished (see Cathy Morley's chapter in this book). Thus, trying to achieve a balance of knowledge sharing can be difficult. Conventional dietetics often suffers from the problem of unhinging itself from earlier ties to home economics. Legacies of early days are often seen to be a disadvantage because of the similarities with housework and other forms of labour which in the eyes of some have low status. The 'scientific turn' in dietetics, marked by training in universities, adoption of the scientific method and the emulation of various markers of biomedicine – research, conferences, scientific journals, etc. – all of which were believed to give prestige to the discipline, meant that cookery, cuisine and gastronomy took a back seat. Yet we can now see that to be fully effective, training in and appreciation of the culinary arts are vital for the translation of nutritional science into foods, meals and other forms of alimentation into the habits of people. We can appreciate this in the stories of Katy and Louis, already told above, where each of our actors is applying their own understanding of what is 'good' to eat.

Conclusion

The purpose of this chapter is to highlight the different understandings of ethics in dietetic practice that goes beyond the traditional role of protecting the interests of patients and communities. As is clear in the scenarios painted in this chapter, different forms of knowledge are culturally bound and historically and traditionally situated. In appreciating these differences, dietitians have to steer a careful course between the scientistic foundations that are obviously important in dietetic practices; there is no room for an 'anything goes', laissez-faire approach. But neither should the dominance of bioscience rule what dietitians offer to their patients and communities. Where does critical dietetics help here? The multidisciplinarity that welcomes multiple understandings of knowledge, tradition and empiricism allows a nuanced appreciation of practice. But there are some obvious potholes. Critical dietetics, as a nascent movement, will undoubtedly encounter misunderstandings and misconceptions. One inevitable problem concerns a failure to appreciate the aims and ambitions of critical dietetics, believing it to be a rebuke of conventional dietetics rather than as a different way of thinking. As such, critical dietetics may be accused of being revolutionary rather than evolutionary, rebellious rather than radical and belligerent rather than progressive. In short, critical dietetics will no doubt experience many of the criticisms that have been levelled at movements striving to encourage new thinking in areas of conventional thinking and practice.

Finally, as a bioscience, conventional dietetics generates knowledge informed by the so-called scientific method. This is chiefly concerned with the collection of facts through experimental observations to test hypotheses. Facts are seen to be 'out there', awaiting discovery and external to human consciousness; as such, the 'objects' of dietetic knowledge are often rendered universal, stable in time and space and inanimate. This assumption is applied as much to human subjects, eating environments and human relationships, as to food constituents. However, as mentioned earlier, critical dietetics sees facts and their meanings to be constructed within particular cultures and traditions. The rise and fall of particular meanings about facts are part of scientific and political discourses. If this is correct, then the role of ethics in dietetics practices becomes even more important. That is to say, if it is accepted that facts and their meanings are socially and culturally constructed, then 'eating right' becomes a contested space. Critical dietetics is set to explore that space.

Assignments

1. Students will examine the food habits and food choices of two different cultures. They will explore and explain different assumptions about what foods are 'good' to eat and what foods are restricted. Students will explain the roles of science and of tradition in explaining why foods are categorised as good or not good to eat.
2. Students will discuss the ethical dilemmas associated with the following scenario. Julian is a dietitian in a children's hospital situated in a large city. Recently a 3-year-old girl has been admitted with frank malnutrition and wasting. It appears that the child has been raised on a strict vegan diet that her parents have been following for many years. The parents have been asking why their child has not been growing well, especially given the obvious advantages of the natural diet they have been following. Julian has been asked to meet and talk with the parents to provide answers to their questions.

Definition of Keywords and Terms

Disenchantment	The move away from more mystical forms of belief towards a rational, secular approach to organising social groups. In this context the term owes an intellectual debt to nineteenth-century sociologist, Max Weber, who employed the term to explain the move in western cultures towards bureaucratic and modernised forms of rationalism.
Epistemology	The study of knowledge and its creation and justification. In this chapter epistemology has been explored through the ways in which knowledge is culturally and historically created.
Ethics	Principles that govern behaviour that have a strong moral foundation.
Gastronomy	The appreciation of the art and knowledge of food and cooking. In this chapter, gastronomic has been used to refer to the use of senses and experience in food choice.
Ontology	A philosophical term referring to the way things exist or are being. In this chapter the term is used to highlight the ways in which food and nourishment support growth and development of physical things (bodies) but also abstract things like mental and spiritual existence.
Scientism	A belief that science and the scientific method is the only way of understanding natural or social phenomena. This chapter has used the term scientistic to refer to a preference for scientific method and proof.

How This Chapter Addresses the Critical Dietetics Framework

This chapter has addressed the following elements of the framework:

An appreciation of multidisciplinary and trans-theoretical approaches to understanding food, health and people. This means that conventional wisdom in dietetics, which is often rooted in biosciences, is complemented by scholarship in the social sciences and the humanities. The resulting larger body of knowledge allows for a richer insight into the problems that dietetics and nutritional sciences are required to address.

The chapter positions dietetic practices as being not only bioscientific but informed by concepts in the social sciences and humanities. In particular the social and cultural construction of knowledge and belief systems demonstrates an appreciation of a trans-theoretical approach.

A belief that policy and practice positions should be socially just and, as such, socially accountable to those who are expected to be benefited from the actions of dietetics and nutrition science.

In privileging different ways of knowing food health and bodies, the chapter takes into account the various positions from which people speak, including those whose voices would otherwise not be heard.

References

Coveney J (2006) Food, morals and meaning: the pleasure and anxiety of eating, 2nd edn. Routledge, London

Coveney J (2014) Food. Routledge, London

Crotty P (1995) Good nutrition?: fact and fashion in dietary advice. Allen and Unwin, Sydney

Elliott A (2001) Concepts of the self. Polity Press, Cambridge

Petersen A (2007) The body in question: a socio-cultural approach. Routledge, London

Reiger K (1985) The disenchantment of the home: modernising the Australian family 1880–1940. Oxford University Press, Melbourne

Chapter 9
Food, Dietetics, and Imperialism

Jill H. White

Aim of Chapter and Learning Outcomes

The aim of this chapter is to expose the readers to the concept that we live in a system where food is produced for profit instead of meeting people's nutrition and health needs and respecting the Earth.

After reading this chapter, readers will:

(i) Identify the role of profit in food production, distribution, and quality.
(ii) Analyze the historical role class, race, gender, and war have played in agriculture and food access.

Summary

Through a critical lens, we will trace the history of food production, the growth of the food and grocery industries. We will discuss the effects of war and government policy in collusion with Western agricultural conglomerates that have resulted in unfair trade agreements, leading to mass migration and the destruction of local agricultural communities. Race, class, and gender oppressions, resulting in the global povertization of women and children, intersect with safe food and water access. Our hope is to talk about people struggling for food justice and alternative systems that will inspire readers to become advocates for equal access to healthy food, healthcare, education, and environmental consciousness for all.

J. H. White (✉)
Nutrition Science, Dominican University, River Forest, IL, USA
e-mail: jwhite@dom.edu

© Springer Nature Switzerland AG 2019
J. Coveney, S. Booth (eds.), *Critical Dietetics and Critical Nutrition Studies*,
Food Policy, https://doi.org/10.1007/978-3-030-03113-8_9

Introduction

I often begin my courses by asking students: What is the goal of the food industry in the United States? Is it to feed people? No, the goal of the food and agricultural industries is to make money. We live in the economic system of capitalism, where food (and healthcare, along with most goods and services) is for profit, not for sustaining people or the environment. We are now in the stage of capitalism called imperialism.

Imperialism is the final stage of capitalism that is reached when the capitalists of a particular country are compelled to economically expand beyond their own borders through military force or other methods of coercion. Imperialism is referred to as the highest stage of capitalism because the capitalist system must either expand or die in its quest to accumulate profits. Vladimir Lenin was a leader of the 1917 Bolshevik Revolution in Russia and a prominent Marxist who popularized the term "imperialism" and provided it with a scientific definition. Lenin identified five essential features of imperialism in his germinal work on the subject, "Imperialism: The Highest Stage of Capitalism." The five features of imperialism are (1) the creation of decisive monopolies through the concentration of production and capital; (2) the merger of bank capital and industrial capital to create an oligarchy of financial capital; (3) the export of capital and commodities, with capital being the more fundamental of the two; (4) the formation of global capitalist monopolies that share the world among themselves; and (5) the territorial division of the whole world among the most powerful capitalist powers (Katz 2001). Does any of this sound familiar today?

For millions of years, humans lived communally, sharing resources, child-rearing, and housing, generally under a matriarchal system. If you look at a yardstick of human history, most of it would be this way, and only a few inches would represent society organized under private property. With the domestication of animals and development of agriculture, humans were then able to produce more than they needed. This was the beginning of class society, the accumulation of wealth and its distribution. Mother right was eventually overturned, and women and children became property of men, who traditionally had been responsible for food production and instrumentation.

All class society is characterized by exploitation—whether under feudalism or under semifeudal chattel slave conditions like in the United States, where enslaved Africans had no rights and all they produced belonged to the master. A profit system cannot exist without exploitation; it is the source of profit. Class society is divided between the ruling class, who own and control the wealth and resources, and the working class, who are actually the majority of society. The ruling class controls the means of production (factories, etc.) and repressive forces of the state apparatus (police, military, etc.) to maintain power. They invented racism, sexism, and other forms of oppression and repression to divide the working class to keep them from uniting to demand their rightful portion. The "class struggle" is really the struggle between the tiny ruling class and the majority working class over who controls the profits of society. It is the 1% versus the 99%.

History of the Food Industry

Capitalism emergence out of the medieval world reveals a basic process that is fundamental to understanding why we have a food system that fails so many individuals and communities. This process is one of dispossession—stripping people of the means to independently provide for themselves and their community. Dispossession of land access is the first step, but the process continues over access to tools, materials, knowledge, and, ultimately, time (Tarr 2013).

The scientific revolution provided tools and ways of thinking that increased production. Improved transportation and industry allowed for a global economy—the most famous aspect being the triangle trade route between Europe, Africa, and the New World, with its infamous middle passage. Europeans seized land from the native people and occupied it. Globalized production and trade gave new life to the institution of slavery, which created one of the dominant forms of American agriculture, and its social and cultural order. In the nineteenth century, the factory system arose in the North, the plantation system was solidified throughout the South, and vast fields of grain production were opened up in the rich virgin lands of the Midwest. These activities were facilitated by gains in technological knowledge: the cotton gin, advances in coal and steam power, better plows, textile factory machinery, steamboats, railroads, mechanical harvesters and threshers, and large-scale grain elevators. With an expanded market and longer supply lines, food systems became less regional or local (Tarr 2013).

The modern food economy was increasingly national in scope with the rail system, new refrigerated cars, and publically subsidized water projects. Meat production was dominated by the huge stockyards and packing houses like Swift and Armour. Prices for all foodstuffs were now nationally set instantaneously, via the telegraph. Industrial agriculture had arrived.

The great depression was first felt in the farm sector, well before the stock market crash. Farming was plagued by problems of overproduction and underconsumption. The political power of farm states and the devastation of rural communities in the 1930s as families were driven off farms all contributed to the passage of the first comprehensive farm programs, which remained in place in one form or another until the 1970s. The industrialization and consolidation of agriculture continued as more and more food firms became vertically integrated (one company controlling several steps in the production process, for instance, an oil company owning refineries and gas stations) (Tarr 2013).

In the early 1970s, the Nixon administration made a major change to federal farm programs that had a significant effect. The essence of it was the Secretary of Agriculture Earl Butz's statement to farmers to "get big or get out." Farmers, now calling themselves agribusinessmen, took out huge debt loads to buy more land and ever-larger and more expensive machinery to work it.

Today the US food system is fully industrialized. Large agribusiness corporations dominate agriculture. Just three or four large companies handle almost all grain in the United States. The industry is rapidly consolidating and centralizing—

from seeds to grocery store. A few giant corporations control the vast majority of a particular market (Tarr 2013).

As one observer noted, "Capitalism presents us with the paradoxical reality of a rapid growth of food production and perpetuation of overproduction (relative to markets and income distributions) on the one hand, accompanied by the reinforcement of social exclusion and thus the growth of hunger on the other" (Pollan 2008).

End of Family Farming

Agricultural resources and enhanced techniques allowed food prices to drop. This was great for the consumer but bad for the small farmers' income. The government subsidized commodities programs, benefitting large agribusiness. Large food companies receive 20% return on their investments. Only 3–5% on investments are received by even the top third of family farmers. The decline in family farms has changed the format of the socioeconomic status of rural America.

In the rest of the world, the process of capital accumulation and dispossession grinds on: small farmers continue to be driven off the land and into the urban slums of the underdeveloped world. This is in no small part due to the actions of the developed and wealthy world. One such action is American subsidies to domestic growers, which allows them to export the flood of surplus to developing countries, thus undercutting and eventually destroying local producers. The relentless downward pressure on wages since the 1970s has more than anything been responsible for "economic growth" over the past 40 years. The effect has been the necessity for more Americans to work longer hours and to look for less expensive options in things such as food (Tarr 2013).

Grocery Industry

After World War II ended, supermarket expansion picked up. Many small independent grocers were driven out of business and bought out by larger corporations. By 1977, there was a 40,000 square foot Piggly Wiggly similar to that of a modern-day superstore Walmart. It had an in-store bakery, a sit-down eating areas, and a flower shop. A new format, the big-box store, began to compete in food sales. By 2002 Walmart surpassed Kroger to become the largest US chain and increased its worldwide food grocery business to become the largest in the world. Walmart's expansion outside the United States and the entry of other international players led to the already globalized supply chains' greater reliance on distant sources. Food retailers have increasingly focused on food marketing, emphasizing the messages associated with food products rather than the nutritional content of the foods themselves. This trend has intensified the tendency toward the increased processing, reformulation of products, and use of varied packaging for improved marketing. Products such as sodas, sugary cereals, candy, and potato chips are made affordable, even as the increased portion sizes of such products offer far less nutritional value per calorie provided. Thus, supermarkets have become one more contributor to changes in diet and health and have increased trends toward unhealthy eating, particularly in low-income communities (Gottlieb and Joshi 2013). The grocery industry may now come full cycle with the rising popularity of home-delivered goods.

Race, Class, and Food Access

The absence of full-service markets and limited food choices available in low-income communities are crucial food justice issues. A study published in the *Journal of Preventive Medicine* examined the availability of supermarkets, grocery stores, and convenience stores in the United States (Bower et al. 2014). Data obtained from the 2000 census bureau and 2001 InfoUSA revealed that as neighborhood poverty increased, supermarket availability decreased. Regardless of poverty status, Black neighborhoods had the fewest supermarkets, while white neighborhoods had the most. Data was analyzed from similar sociodemographic census block groups and 1953 supermarkets across the United States. Associations were made between the socioeconomic status of neighborhoods and the proportion of Black and/or Hispanic population with the prices of healthy and unhealthy foods. It was found that consistently, across all neighborhood characteristics, the price of healthier foods was just about twice as high as the price of unhealthy foods (Kern et al. 2017). A study published in the *American Journal of Health Promotion* in September of 2016 explored the pricing and availability of foods and beverages specifically in the Navajo populations across the nation. What was found was that the Navajo convenience stores offered less healthy food options than the supermarkets. In both types of stores, the healthier food items identified were all more expensive than their corresponding, less healthy versions.

Trade Agreements Destroy Local Agriculture

NAFTA became a symbol of Mexico's growing economic dependence on the United States because corn is not only a staple of the Mexican diet but also a symbol of Mexico itself. As recently as the early 1980s, Mexico exported surplus corn but now buys a third of the corn it consumes from the United States, making Mexico the largest corn export market for US farmers. Since NAFTA's implementation, Mexico's annual per capita growth flatlined to one of the lowest in the hemisphere, real wage declined, and unemployment went up. Mexican producer's prices fell, and small farmers found themselves unable to make a living; hence many were forced to leave their farms. At the same time, consumer food prices rose. Under NAFTA, the capitalist government of Mexico agreed to withdraw long-standing price supports, credit, and technical assistance for Mexican peasants. Meanwhile, corn and beans were being subsidized in the United States and shipped south. US corn was sold at prices 20–30% below the cost of production. Two million farmers in Mexico were forced to abandon their land. In 1995, 1 year after the implementation of NAFTA, the Mexican peso collapsed from financial speculation in Mexican bonds, primarily by Wall Street sharks. When the Mexican government could not pay the debt on the bonds, the economy collapsed (Goldstein 2008).

War, Forced Migration, and Food Access

According to the World Health Organization (WHO), 65.6 million people were forced to migrate because of war. Migration is the movement from one area to another, and forced migration is the unwilling movement of one area to another. Hunger is related to forced migration. In 2016, it was reported that 100 million people lack food access. The Middle East and North Africa have the largest migrant population. Malnourishment is experienced in conflict areas since crops are destroyed, water is contaminated, food storage are destroyed, and animals and trees are killed. With poor food access, individuals are at higher risk of disease and hunger.

What capitalists call globalization is an expansion of imperialism. Globalization has plunged hundreds of millions of people around the globe into desperate poverty. Although the bosses talk about the modern "peaceful" expansion of capitalism, the reality is that the United States alone has been at war almost every year since the fall of the Soviet Union and has caused the deaths and injuries of millions in imperialist wars since the term "globalization" was popularized (Katz 2001). Now, instead of colonizing oppressed countries through the brute force of imperialist armies alone, bankers and corporations use institutions like the World Bank and the International Monetary Fund to help coerce those countries into bending to their will. Those who try to resist globalization still face the threat of imperialist war. More than a million people were killed by the US-led imperialist coalition against Iraq after Iraq's leaders dared to nationalize their own oil fields and use their resources for the independent development of their own country. The people of Iraq had a total displacement of 4.8 million. It was reported that one-fourth of Iraqi children became malnourished (Mowafi 2011).

Although many jobs have dried up and developed capitalist countries throughout the world no longer seek as much low-wage labor, people from poor countries wracked by misery and war are taking almost unimaginable risks to make their way to developed countries where they hope for a better future. Often, it is to the very imperialist countries whose ruling classes have for generations fattened off exploiting the labor and resources of their homelands. According to the UN High Commissioner on Refugees, in the Central Mediterranean route between Libya and Italy, one person has died for each 47 who made it through.

Worldwide Povertization of Women and Children Effects of Food Access

Women are still the poorest of the poor; among people living in absolute poverty, women make up 70%. Women work two-thirds of all working hours in the world, produce half of the world's food, yet earn only 10% of the world's income and own 1% of property. Of the illiterate adults live in the world, two-thirds of them are women (Yehya and Dutta 2015).

Experts at the International Labour Organization noted that discrimination and exploitation of women are gradually increasing in the twenty-first century. It is women who suffer most from cuts in government social programs, unemployment, and worsening job conditions. The average level of their wages is 30% less than men—even in the most developed economies of Europe and the United States.

At the same time, it should be remembered that the problems of women from Third World countries are much more serious and bigger than in developed countries, as transnational corporations move production to the periphery, actively using cheap female labor. In Europe and the United States, there is also a gender gap, but in poor countries, whose super-exploitation is the basis of First World prosperity, the situation of women is truly disastrous. This includes meager salaries, underpaid and forced labor without proper conditions of job safety, and lack of maternity leave—and, consequently, of the ability to take care of children, who often suffer from hunger.

Women and children are most vulnerable to the effects of poverty. Children raised in low-income families have higher risk of malnutrition, increased exposure to environmental toxins, impaired cognitive development, lead poisoning, and obesity. Over one billion people worldwide are undernourished, and global studies indicate that malnutrition in pre-/postnatal periods of life is closely linked to developmental delays (Yehya and Dutta 2015).

Children from low-income families are often behind in school. Eighty percent are so far behind that they are unable to read proficiently by the end of third grade, and students who are not able to master reading by that time are 13 times more likely to drop out of school (Masuku-Maseko and Owaga 2012). In the United States, it is estimated that one in four children under the age of 6 lives in home struggling with poverty. Comparatively one in four children in Africa goes hungry (Masuku-Maseko and Owaga 2012). Food insecurity holds different obstacles depending on the geographical region. In America, food insecurity is commonly seen with food deserts and limited access to fresh food. Countries worldwide are facing concerns of food insecurity from climate change, drought, massive flooding or war, and dislocation.

In America, many women report working more than one shift in a single day at work and barely getting by. In the workplace, low-income women are viewed as disposable and easily replaced by other low-income women. Because of this, women are more likely to experience anxiety and depression due to fear of being let go as well as from financial stress. New mothers may be afraid of losing their job, so they may not take their full maternity leave, leading to additional stress. Parents may reduce or eliminate their own meal to give their child more food. This may lead to malnutrition and perhaps other nutrition-related diseases of the mother.

Health and Environmental Effects of Western Food System

Globalization of Fast Food

The United States is an industrialized country with high rates of nutrition-related diseases affecting both adults and children. It is possible to eat and still be malnourished; not all foods will properly fuel our bodies, and unfortunately fast food provides poor-quality food in mass to low-income neighborhoods. By this logic, the fast-food industry has contributed to the development of food deserts and undernourished diets worldwide.

Fast-food menu options vary from country to country. Each restaurant is tailored to meet and exceed the culture of the geographical region. In the article, "Exposing Diabetes Mellitus to Asia, The Impact of Western-Style Fast Food," researchers reviewed the correlation between fast-food eating and health risks (Pan et al. 2012). Using a Singapore-Chinese study, over 43,000 individuals participated and were followed for 5 years. Results indicated that individuals who ate fast food twice per week were at a 27% increase risk of developing type 2 diabetes. Furthermore, the risk of developing and mortality from coronary heart disease was 56% higher than those who ate little-to-no fast food.

In El Salvador, a study was performed to find the relationship between advertisement and consumption of fast food. "An interpretive Study of Food, Snack, and Beverage Advertisements in Rural and Urban El Salvador" is an article that looks into the various technique advertisements used to draw in viewers to a specific product. El Salvador is a country that faces health disparities, low/middle income, and malnutrition. However, there has been a sudden increase in overweight/obesity due to changes in individual's diet (Amanzadeh et al. 2015). With advertisements playing a key role in the success of fast-food restaurants, photographic data was collected from six rural villages. One hundred different advertisements for fast food, beverages, and snack were taken. In the 1990s, Thailand was considered a developing country that faced undernutrition. However, with the emergence of fast-food restaurants, a new health threat appeared. Overweight and obesity became more common in the population's health. The traditional food found seen in this country consisted of rice, vegetable dishes, and fish. This diet was low in fat. However, with fast food present in the country, there was a shift in the population's diet. There was an increase in the consumption of oil and animal fat and a decrease in vegetables and fruit.

Environmental Implications

Environmental changes that negatively impact the food systems, particularly in developing countries, are expected to destabilize the global food systems over time. The three recurring themes that relate climate change and food systems include vulnerability and adaptation, sustainable food systems, and biophysical impacts on food production.

Each sector of the current food system has an effect on the environment. The degree of these effects depends on a variety of natural and human-driven processes. For example, the increasing use of mineral fertilizers has created growth in productivity in the US agriculture over the past 50 years; however, it has also caused negative effects to the environment such as greenhouse gas (GHG) emissions and a decrease in water quality. GHG emissions can be the result of burning fossil fuels in the food manufacturing process during food distributions. Food losses are estimated to contribute to 1.4 kg of carbon dioxide equivalent to the carbon footprint of the US average diet. This is the equivalent to 33 million vehicles yearly. Beef accounts for only 4% of the retail food supply by weight and is 36% of the diet-related GHG emissions (Heller and Keoleian 2015).

The Flint Water Crisis: Environmental Racism

Lead can cause immediate acute poisoning. Exposure in young children can lead to diminished or loss in intelligence, development, behavior, attention, and other neurological functions. Children who are exposed to high levels of lead are at risk of anemia and decreased bone and muscle growth, as well as damage to the reproductive organs and nervous system. Lead poisoning can permanently alter human DNA. Those that suffer from lead poisoning might also pass the health conditions that they developed to their children and grandchildren.

In April 2014, the city of Flint in Michigan switched its water supply from the Detroit water supply to a new water supplier, Karegnondi Water Authority (KWA), to cut costs and save the city from financial collapse. However, KWA was still in the process of constructing their pipelines, and completion of the work was not scheduled until 2016. As a result, Flint officials decided to use the Flint River water as an alternative source in the meantime. As soon as the switched was made, residents started complaining about the odor, taste, and smell of the water that is coming out of their faucets. Residents also complained about getting rashes, losing hair, or becoming more ill due to the water. Water tests revealed high levels of chlorination by-product trihalomethane (TTHM), which is linked to cancer and other associated health problems. To kill off the harmful bacteria in the water, city officials issued advisories to the residents of Flint to boil their water. City officials also claimed their water was safe to drink. In 2015, researchers tested Flint's water and found high levels of lead in the city's drinking water. Similarly, a pediatrician tested the children's blood and found high levels of lead. A federal state of emergency was declared in 2016.

This is a prime example of environmental injustice. According to the United States Environmental Protection Agency (EPA), environmental justice is defined as the fair treatment and meaningful involvement of all people regardless of race, color, national origin, or income, with respect to the development, implementation, and enforcement of environmental laws, regulations, and policies. But this is not the case in Flint where the population is predominantly African American with a low socioeconomic background. African Americans are disproportionately exposed to polluted air, water, and soil. Many believed that race and social class were the main reasons why the local and state governments' response were extremely slow. Reports of chemical compounds exceeding the federally allowable levels were recorded; however government officials claimed that it was not a top health concern and the issue would fade away eventually. Michigan health department issued a report that states the Flint water was safe.

Exploited Food Workers

Social inequality is basic to the operations within the farming industry and food industry as evidenced by the lack of resources and opportunities for food workers, starting from the farm enterprise to the food retailer. The union between the farming industry and food industry invigorates the agro-food chain. Since policy-makers' primary goal is to uphold the economy, many have sacrificed individuals' livelihoods to maintain power and financial wealth.

US growers recruit the hardest working and most vulnerable workers to maximize profits. Since the wages in the United States are nearly ten times higher than in Mexico and guest workers' legal status is tentative, they feel they have no other alternative to earn a living for themselves and their families. Growers exploit guest workers by paying them less than minimum wage while demanding production to exceed 10 h/day over 5 days/week.

Researchers examined the correlation between workplace and housing conditions and farmworkers' usage of pesticide practices and Personal Protective Equipment (PPE) (Levesque et al. 2012). During the agricultural growing season (July to October 2010) in Stokes, Yadkin, Surry, and Rowan counties in North Carolina, farmworkers aged 18–62 years completed a questionnaire on housing and workplace conditions. Despite the US Environmental Protection Agency Worker Protection Standard (EPA WPS) and Occupational Safety and Health Administration (OSHA) establishing sanitary field regulations for nonhazardous and healthy work conditions, farmworkers and their families are inflicted significantly by pesticide poisoning (Levesque et al. 2012). Abhorrent workplace and housing conditions continue to affect the health of farmworkers. Not only does the United States outsource jobs to foreign companies to maximize profits and give jobs to guest workers who earn paltry wages, but they also automate jobs, invigorating American industries in overseas markets.

Despite the restaurant industry being one of the largest and fastest growing of the US economy, it is still the lowest-paying employer in the US fast food, and full-service restaurants are the least compensated because of the National Restaurant Association's (NRA) leverage and power in Congress. Consequently, approximately six million workers in the United States were legally paid $2.13 per hour in the year 2017. Employees of the food industry are subject to the most sexual harassment compared to other industries in the United States. Research has proven that female-tipped workers were advised by the management to objectify themselves to earn more tips.

Sociologists say fast-food workers are inflicted by "relative deprivation," epitomized by low wages and poor-working conditions (Beaver 2016). This is demonstrated by alienation, paltry wages, wage theft, and the lack of union representation. Many fast-food workers describe their responsibilities of resembling the assembly line nature of work either boring or terrible. In addition, the average hourly median wage for fast-food workers is presently $8.94. To add insult to injury, many fast-food workers are subjected to wage theft as evidenced by not being paid for overtime, being denied mandated breaks, and having hours subtracted from their paychecks. Meanwhile, in the past 15 years, CEOs' compensation of the fast-food industry has quadrupled which is now averaging approximately $22 million per year, while fast-food employees have only been awarded 0.3% increase in their pay (Beaver 2016). The fast-food industry embraces the "family" culture to suppress unions in order to maintain obedience, which is the most valued characteristic in the fast-food crew. But brave workers from the food industry, primarily those from immigrant communities, have led the struggle for unionization and $15 minimum living wage in the United States.

An Alternative Food System

With the collapse of the Soviet Union and the tightening of the US embargo, the early 1990s saw Cuba facing a severe food crisis and a collapse of more than 30% of the island's GDP. Cubans were forced to develop a new method of farming: urban agriculture. Citizens used balconies, backyards, and roof terraces for cultivation and raising livestock. Rural farmers adopted agroecological methods due to the lack of oil-based pesticides and fertilizers. Organic principles were followed, and locally available resources were used. They practiced crop rotation and intercropping, used green manure, and planted hedges. Using repellent plants such as common thyme, basil, marigold, maize, or ruddles, they effectively reduced pest infestation and attracted beneficial insects. It turned out to be a model of food production that guarantees the preservation of natural resources and relies on minimum artificial inputs, from a sustainable perspective (Iozzi 2016).

A cornerstone of agroecology is diversification of both crops and farming methods—including livestock integration—that contributes to the promotion of biodiversity and of a more efficient use of resources, such as sunlight, water, soil, and natural pests. This effort rendered the island a world leader in sustainable agriculture, and its food production system became a model for other countries in the world to follow, especially developing societies that should be guarded against any damaging transformations.

According to the World Wildlife Fund (WWF) biannual Living Planet Report 2016, Cuba is the most sustainable country on the planet. Indeed, the fund created an environmental footprint index that combines the human development and the exploitation of natural resources. The island was found to have both an acceptable ecological footprint per capita, using an exemplary amount of energy and natural resources, and an acceptable Human Development Index rating. Such indicators demonstrate that a sustainable system of food production is compatible with a high level of literacy, life expectancy, and low infant mortality. According to the data collected by the Food and Agriculture Organization (FAO), some 795 million people in the world do not have enough food to lead a healthy active life—about one in nine people on Earth. This is a clear indication that the promotion of industrial agriculture has failed to deliver satisfactory results. Industrial food systems affect human health and broader ecological systems.

A sustainable agricultural model, such as the Cuban one, may be looked at as an alternative to improve food security and environment health. Cuba's urban agriculture has become a model for the rest of developing world. Cuba has a socialist political system in which property rights and agricultural policies, as well as healthcare, are managed in a centralized way, significantly different from the rest of the world. This food production represents an alternative for countries fighting hunger to be able to assure the necessary sustenance to their own population and an opportunity for everyone to live in a sustainable world. It is a system that puts people and care of the Earth before profits and assures food and health as a basic human right.

Conclusion

A critical examination of the food supply demonstrates that food production, and the development of food industries, allows an examination of the ways in which vested interests can sway a government policy and market forces. The total effect has been a global povertization of women and children, intersect with safe food and water access. We are now better aware of people struggling for food justice and alternative systems. Examining the journey of countries like Cuba gave us the opportunity to see how sustainability can be achieved. The question is: How can we use this knowledge to better food systems everywhere?

Acknowledgments I would like to thank and recognize the contribution of graduate students from Dominican University Fall 2017 Food and Social Justice class for their assistance in providing information for this paper, a proof again that seeking knowledge is always a collective activity, not a private property.

Assignments

1. Select a community that appears to have a population at nutrition risk, and complete a Nutrition Community Assessment. Include the following:

   Location
   Demographics of the population
   State of nutrition/major health issues of the community/neighborhood area
   Grocery stores in community/neighborhood
   Food pantries and depositories in community/neighborhood
   Food support agency (WIC, Food Stamps) that would address nutrition/health concerns for children and families that might be helpful

2. Grocery Store Assessment
   Take a look at the document linked below, so you are aware of this kind of review. Print pages 158–160, and do a grocery store review of either a store in the neighborhood assessed or another neighborhood grocery store somewhere different than where you live. Just write down prices (lowest-cost item in this category). Write a one-page reflection of the experience. Does it allow consumers to apply the Thrifty Food Plan? What was the atmosphere, clean, efficient, or chaotic? Would you shop here or recommend it to family and friends?

3. Research a movement to fight health/food disparity. Write a two-page report.

4. Develop goals and outreach materials for a Food is a Right Movement activity.

Definition of Keywords and Terms

Agribusiness	It is the business of agricultural production. The term was coined in 1957 by Goldberg and Davis. It includes agrichemicals, breeding, crop production (farming and contract farming), distribution, farm machinery, processing, and seed supply, as well as marketing and retail sales. All agents of the food and fiber value chain and those institutions that influence it are part of the agribusiness system.
Capitalism	A system of economics based on the private ownership of capital and production inputs and on the production of goods and services for profit.
Class society	The Communist Manifesto describes the process by which society developed over time, so today it is divided into roughly two great classes. Marxists often refer to the ruling class as the bourgeoisie

	and the working class as the proletariat. Each class is defined by its relationship to the major means of production.
Globalization	Bosses and bourgeois politicians talk about globalization as if it is a new and benign form of capitalism that peacefully spreads wealth and stability to poor countries around the world. But the truth is that what the mainstream media calls globalization is just a modern form of imperialism. Now, instead of colonizing oppressed countries through the brute force of imperialist armies alone, bankers and corporations use institutions like the World Bank and the International Monetary Fund to help coerce those countries into bending to their will.
Imperialism	Imperialism is the final stage of capitalism that is reached when the capitalists of a particular country are compelled to economically expand beyond their own borders through military force or other methods of coercion.
NAFTA	The *North American Free Trade Agreement* is an agreement signed by Canada, Mexico, and the United States, creating a trilateral trade bloc in North America.

How This Chapter Addresses the Critical Dietetic Framework

A belief that policy and practice positions should be socially just and, as such, socially accountable to those who are expected to be benefited from the actions of dietetics and nutrition science.

The goal of this chapter was to expose the readers to the concept that we live in a system where food is produced for profit instead of meeting people's nutrition and health needs and respecting the Earth. Through a critical lens, we traced the history of food production and the growth of the food and grocery industries. We discussed the effects of war and government policy in collusion with Western agricultural conglomerates that have resulted in unfair trade agreements, leading to the mass migration and the destruction of local agricultural communities. Race, class, and gender oppressions have resulted in the global povertization of women and children and intersect with safe food and water access. Our hope is to inspire readers to become advocates for equal access to healthy food, healthcare, education, and environmental consciousness for all.

References

Amanzadeh B, Sokal-Gutierrez K, Barker JC (2015) An interpretive study of food, snack and beverage advertisements in rural and urban El Salvador. BMC Public Health 15(1):521. https://doi.org/10.1186/s12889-015-1836-9

Beaver W (2016) Fast-food unionization. Society 53(5):469–473

Bower K, Thorpe R, Rohde C et al (2014) The intersection of neighborhood racial segregation, poverty, and urbanicity and its impact on food store availability in the United States. Prev Med 58:33–39

Goldstein F (2008) Low-wage capitalism. World View Forum, New York

Gottlieb R and Joshi A (2013) Food justice MIT Press, Cambridge Mass

Heller M, Keoleian G (2015) Greenhouse gas emission estimates of U.S. dietary choices and food loss. J Ind Ecol 19(3):391–401

Katz A (ed) (2001) What is Marxism all about? World View Forum, New York

Kern D, Auchincloss A, Stehr M et al (2017) Healthy and unhealthy food prices across neighborhoods and their association with neighborhood socioeconomic status and proportion Black/Hispanic. J Urban Health 94(4):494–505

Levesque D, Arif A, Shen J (2012) Association between workplace and housing conditions and use of pesticide safety practices and personal protective equipment among North Carolina farmworkers in 2010. Int J Occup Environ Med 3(2):53–67

Iozzi D (2016) Cuba, a model of sustainable agriculture towards global food security coha@coha.org

Masuku-Maseko S, Owaga E (2012) Child malnutrition and mortality in Swaziland: situation analysis of the immediate, underlying and basic causes. Afr J Food Agric Nutr Dev 12(2):5994–6006

Mowafi H (2011) Conflict, displacement and health in the Middle East. Global Public Health 6:472–487

Pan A, Malik VS, Hu FB (2012) Exporting diabetes mellitus to Asia: the impact of western-style fast food. Circulation 126(2):163–165. https://doi.org/10.1161/circulationaha.112.115923

Pollan M (2008) In defense of food: an eater's manifesto. Penguin Press, New York

Tarr S (2013) Food and social justice. In: White J (ed) Diversity and disparity in nutrition education http://dom.constellation.libras.org/handle/10969/9111

Yehya N, Dutta M (2015) Articulations of health and poverty among women on WIC. Health Commun 30(12):1223–1233

Chapter 10
Social Justice, Health Equity, and Advocacy: What Are Our Roles?

Jennifer Brady

Aim of Chapter and Learning Outcomes

The aims of this chapter are:

- To explore literature on health and social justice, health equity, health advocacy, and health activism
- To explore the dietetic profession's and dietetic practitioners' engagement in social justice advocacy and health activism
- To explore the opportunities and examples of socially just practice related to food, health, and nutrition

By the end of this chapter, readers will be able to:

- Discuss key terms including social justice, health equity, health advocacy, and health activism.
- Define and discuss some key terms related to health advocacy and activism including intersectionality, health equity, social justice, healthism, and nutritionism.
- Discuss the importance of dietitians' roles in health advocacy.
- Identify specific examples of dietitians' involvement in health advocacy.

J. Brady (✉)
Mount Saint Vincent University, Halifax, NS, Canada
e-mail: Jennifer.Brady@msvu.ca

© Springer Nature Switzerland AG 2019   143
J. Coveney, S. Booth (eds.), *Critical Dietetics and Critical Nutrition Studies*,
Food Policy, https://doi.org/10.1007/978-3-030-03113-8_10

Summary

This chapter explores social justice, health equity, and advocacy, with a view to demonstrate the ways in which dietitians may take up roles to advance social justice. The chapter will review literature on social justice, health equity, and health advocacy from across various health (i.e. social work, nursing) and non-health professions (i.e. urban planning, architecture, library sciences), as well as literature specific to dietetic knowledge and practice. To end, interviews with social justice advocates and activists are included as case studies to illustrate advocacy in different areas of dietetic practice.

Introduction

Do dietitians have a role to play in advancing social justice through advocacy and activism? If so, what roles might they play? What issues might dietitians seek to address? How might dietitians join others who are already involved in social justice movements? This chapter seeks to explore these questions in light of the dramatic social, economic, and environmental shifts that threaten the health and well-being of populations across the globe and the growing social movements that have arisen to address them.

In recent years, the world has witnessed ever-worsening income disparities alongside growing racial and gender inequities, threats to national and international peace, and the now evident impacts of climate change on the security of our land, water, and food systems. The collective impact of these phenomena on human health is unmistakable. However, the adverse effects of these phenomena are not equally felt among diverse communities, populations, and regions of the world. Rather, the consequences, particularly for health, are disproportionately shouldered by the economically deprived regions of the world that have long suffered the effects of colonialism, and by the marginalized communities that bear income, racial, and gender inequities across the globe. In short, those who have already been subjugated to economic and social deprivation as a result of social injustices stand to endure the worst of the changes yet to come, including the greatest losses to their health and well-being. It is in this light that I pose the questions that begin this chapter and explore dietitians' roles as advocates in advancing social justice and health equity.

This chapter unfolds in three sections. In the first section, I explore key terms including social justice, health equity, and advocacy. The second section comprises two case studies, each of which includes a conversation between myself and one individual whose work in health, nutrition, food, eating, and bodies is rooted in health equity and social justice. In the third section, I offer some concluding remarks. Ultimately, my hope for this chapter is to inspire individual dietetic practitioners and the collective dietetic profession to embrace roles in health equity advocacy.

Key Concepts

In this section, I discuss key terms, namely, social justice, health equity, and advocacy that are central to the objectives and learning outcomes of this chapter. Rather than providing a singular definition of each term, I endeavour to discuss and demonstrate the complexity of these terms as concepts that comprise multiple and evolving meanings. Appreciating the complexity of these terms is important in thinking through the similarly complex matter of professions' and practitioners' roles in advancing social justice and health equity through advocacy.

Social Justice and Health Equity

Social justice is a concept that evades a singular, unequivocal definition. As Sandretto et al. (2007) note, defining social justice is "a bit like trying to nail jello to the wall, a sticky and difficult task" (p. 308). The multiple facets, priorities, and approaches that may make something socially just, or that may ameliorate inequities that result from injustices, are highly contextual, contested, and sometimes contradictory. Understanding what social justice is, what it looks like, and how to achieve it, therefore, is best done by considering the multiplicity of its meaning and "our often taken-for-granted conceptualizations" of the term (Sandretto et al. 2007, p. 308).

With the need to understand the multiplicity of social justice in mind, I include the following definitions from authors writing from the perspective of various health and non-health professions, including nursing, social work, teacher education, archival science, and public health:

> ...the **fair distribution of society's benefits, responsibilities, and their consequences**... focuses on the relative position of one social group in relationship to others and on the root causes of disparities and what can be done to eliminate them. (Canadian Nurses Association 2010)

> ...full participation in society and the **balancing of benefits and burdens by all citizens, resulting in equitable living and a just ordering of society**. (Buettner-Schmidt and Lobo 2012)

> ...fostering social justice does not simply mean exploring difference or diversity. Rather it uncovers and addresses **systems of power and privilege** that give rise to social inequality...to **critically examine oppression on institutional, cultural, and individual levels**. (Duckworth and Maxwell 2015)

> ...full **human recognition** (disruption of structures of non-recognition; disrespect or marginalization; safety), **fair and just redistribution** (of power; of benefits and burdens; resources, goods and services; wealth; opportunity), **full and equal participation** (in political processes and decision-making; education; employment; community facilities; collective over individual rights; common good), acknowledgement and **remedy historical inequalities** with specific measures (affirmative action; reparations; recognition). (Duff et al. 2013, p. 324)

…refers to the concept of a society that gives individuals and groups **fair treatment and an equitable share of the benefits of society**. In this context, social justice is based on the concepts of **human rights and equity**. Under social justice, all groups and individuals are entitled equally to important rights such as health protection and minimal standards of income. The goal of public health—to minimize preventable death and disability for all—is integral to social justice. (Public Health Agency of Canada 2017)

"**economic, social, and political equity among individuals, groups and institutions**… [and] a necessity of **peace**. (Van Soest 1992)

The definition of social justice inevitably involves a vision of a socially just society in which, among other elements, the **basic needs of all individuals are met** (e.g., material, social-psychological, productive-creative, security, self-actualization and spiritual), **essential institutions are held in public trust** and administered for the good of all in society, work and production reengineered such that individuals are able to integrate their mental, physical and emotional faculties in their work experience, equality of social, civil, cultural and political rights, responsibilities and opportunities exist, and work and products are in harmony with nature. (Birkenmaier 2003)

The lack of definitive definition of social justice may be thought to leave the goals or purpose of social justice advocacy, and therefore dietitians' roles as social justice advocates, ill-defined, directionless, or, worse, immobilized. However, the lack of a concrete definition may also be understood as not only necessary but fruitful. In their work on the politics of local food, DuPuis et al. (2011) devise a notion of "reflexive justice", which they explain is "…a process by which people pursue goals while acknowledging the imperfection of their actions" (p. 297). The authors continue by noting that the process for achieving justice itself is imperfect: "It is also not a particular, fixed, process, but one that responds to changing circumstances, imperfectly, but with an awareness of the contradictions of the moment" (DuPuis et al. 2011, p. 297). For Dupuis, Harrison, and Goodman, the notion of reflexive justice recognizes and works with the complexities and contradictions of social justice in relation to food, eating, and nutrition. For example, the authors describe the tensions between the politics of supporting local food (i.e. campaigns to buy locally grown and produced food that support community-based small business and farmers) and the local inequities related to how that food may be grown (i.e. absent or weak regulation of migrant farm labour and racialized labourers' consequent pesticide exposure). Similarly, Sandretto et al. (2007) note that although democratic decision-making is important, this also must be balanced with measures that avoid fuelling "the tyranny of the majority" that may silence the needs of marginalized groups most affected by an issue but that are fewer in number (p. 316).

What does social justice mean for health and within health professional practice? For some, social justice vis a vis health means simply ensuring "the fair and equal access of all to basic healthcare services and equitable care" (Dharamsi and MacEntee 2002, p. 323). Yet, looking to health care as the means of levelling out health disparities only makes sense if, as Peter (2001) writes, "health care is perceived to be the instrument that is best suited to correct health outcomes" (p. 160). Instead, Peter (2001) and Braveman (2006) argue that increasing access to health care does little to address the myriad social and structural determinants of health, such as income inequity, racism, sexism, colonialism, and so on, that have a greater influence on health than either health care or individual health behaviour (Mikkonen and Raphael 2010). In other words, equitable access to health care is only one necessary precondition for social justice with respect to health, but is not in itself able to ameliorate the underlying causes of the systematically poorer health outcomes experienced by marginalized populations.

How, then, do we conceptualize the pursuit of social justice with respect to health? One answer is health equity[1] (Braveman 2006; Peter 2001). Whitehead (1992) penned one of the most often cited definitions of health equity: "Equity in health implies that ideally everyone should have a *fair opportunity* to attain their full health potential and, more pragmatically, that no one should be disadvantaged from achieving this potential, if it can be avoided" (p. 433). Whitehead (1992) further explains:

> Based on this definition, the aim of policy for equity and health is not to eliminate all health differences so that everyone has the same level and quality of health, but rather to reduce or eliminate those which result from factors that are considered to be both avoidable and unfair. Equity is therefore concerned with creating equal *opportunities* for health, and with bringing health differentials down to the lowest possible level. (p. 434)

Conversely, Whitehead (1992) defines health inequities as "differences in health that are not only unnecessary and avoidable but, in addition, are considered unfair and unjust" (p. 433).

That is, health inequities are not simply a matter of differences in health outcomes, but are caused by avoidable, yet systemic socio-economic disparities that result in poorer health for marginalized populations (Peter 2001).

Dietetics and Social Justice Advocacy

This discussion of social justice and health equity raises further questions about the roles that dietitians might play in ameliorating health inequities. Do dietitians have a role to play in advancing health equity beyond the provision of health services, to acting for structural, systemic change through advocacy? One response to this question may be derived via an emerging framework for health professional education and practice known as "structural competence" (Hansen et al. 2017; Kirmayer et al. 2018; Metzl and Hansen 2014). The notion of structural competence has been developed as a framework for the types of knowledge- and skill-related experiences and abilities that health professionals require to address the underlying causes of health inequities. In contrast to the more commonly used framework of "cultural competence", structural competence calls on professions to address what has been described as the "structural determinants of health" (World Health Organization

---

[1] See Braveman (2006) for an extensive review and discussion of various definitions of health equity.

2010). Addressing equity in mental health and psychiatry professional practice, Metzl and Hansen (2014) explain:

> While cultural competency initiatives train [psychiatry] residents in beliefs and behaviors of patient groups that experience health inequalities, cultural competency often falls short of systemic intervention… The term structural brings into focus institutions and policies that can be altered to promote health equity, while competency signals that there are tangible skills clinicians should acquire to address the social structure factors that act as barriers to improved mental health outcomes. (p. E1)

Translating the knowledge and skills related to structural competence requires that health professionals, including dietitians, engage in advocacy to change policy and engage in action to confront and eliminate social injustices.

Although there are some important texts[2] that address dietitians' roles in redressing the social and structural inequities through advocacy, this pool of literature is small in comparison to that which focuses on nutrition science and individual behaviour change and that within the literatures of other health professions. Hence, several questions remain: What gaps exist in our knowledge, skills, and/or confidence that may prevent us from advocating for change? How, as a profession, might we remedy these potential gaps? What are our current strengths and capacities? How can we respectfully engage with those most impacted by social injustices to learn, listen, and work together for change? The case studies present in the next section shed some light on these questions and point to potential ways forward for dietetics in embracing a role as advocates for social justice and health equity.

Case Studies

The two case studies presented below serve as illustrative examples of the kinds of questions, issues, and conversations that are important to dietitians' engagement in social justice advocacy. Each case study is presented as a conversation[3] between myself (J) and two individuals—Lucy Aphramor (L), a self-identified radical dietitian, performance poet, and founder of *Well Now* located in Coventry, England, and Gloria Lucas (G), an activist and founder of Nalgona Positivity Pride in California, USA. Each conversation unfolds through a series of topic areas that elaborate on Lucy's and Gloria's work, as well as their thoughts about social justice and health equity as these relate to nutrition, food, and health.

---

[2] See, for example, Aphramor et al. (2009), Brady (2017), Raine (2014), Rodriguez (2010), Scott et al. (1998).

[3] The conversations have been edited for readability and to focus the content on the key topics, messages, and insights discussed during the conversation.

Lucy Aphramor

Tell me about your work.

L: There are sort of three main things I do. I train people (people with nutrition or counselling backgrounds, generally), and then I have one-to-one appointments with clients, and I also do poetry.

J: Could you talk a little bit about *Well Now*?

L: I see it as an approach, a starting point for building a fairer world. The starting point is nutrition. My thing is food and bodies. That becomes a vehicle for talking… "tell me your story". If we want change, we have to listen to each other. We have to have a relationship founded on mutual respect. In asking you to tell me your story, what I'm signalling to you is that stories matter, that your experiences matter, that your emotions matter, that knowledge is a co-creation, that I can't just funnel my information into you. It's looking at compassion, curiosity, and connection. Within *Well Now*, that sort of goes into "kindful eating" and "connected eating" and "realistic fitness", the bigger picture of health and body awareness. In order for that to be, it's trauma-informed, compassion-centred, and justice-enhancing. It also has to be relational, body aware, and intentionally political.

J: If someone were to take one of your trainings through *Well Now*, what could they expect?

L: Let's take kindful eating. In a group, the learners themselves have a whole heap of experience. So, we're going to explore that and build on it. The fact that you've come for training implies that there's something else to learn. I'm going to look at what I know; we're going to pool our ideas. What I've learned from my own experiences is that a lot of things that I took in good faith that were presented to me as evidence-based medicine have become taken for granted truths that need challenging. What I've learned about working in trauma and body awareness, to develop an approach and start a conversation, to work with people in a way that asks and questions and helps them figure out things themselves, and to continue your own learning and development. It's not about me transferring facts to you; it's about how this is the start of looking at things differently. And a lot of it is giving people confidence to question the party line and to challenge things.

What does social justice mean to you?

L: At its simplest, it means working in a way that builds a fairer world. So that, for me, means being in the world in a different way than I've been taught as a dietitian. So, what I've sort of figured out working as a dietitian is that socially just practice has to be compassion-centred and trauma-informed in order to be justice-enhancing, and if it's not all three of those, it's none of those. You can't tag on compassion, tag on trauma-informed, you can't tag on social justice— it has to be integrated from the outset. You can't make a neoliberal approach, a social justice approach…. It starts from a very different core set of relational principles.

J: How does that differ from how you were taught? Can you talk about those differences a little bit?

L: What I was taught was a very standard way of approaching health and knowledge and expertise. The implicit assumptions were that there are hierarchies of knowledge where academic knowledge ranks more highly than any other forms of knowledge (particularly, a sort of rarefied academic knowledge that is quantitative), that science is value-free and neutral, that our role as a dietitian is to be an expert, where the dietitian is an expert and the expertise comes from her grasp of scientific knowledge. And the way I was taught had no sense of the role of trauma, the role of body awareness; it was a very mechanical way. And we were taught to think through paradigms that were never meant to include emotions or feelings or humanity or kindness. I had to unlearn a lot of those things.

Also, when we talk about social justice, that for me, we are either using an approach that promotes social justice or social injustice. And so that's not an option! That's not, what I believe, dietitians want to do. We might be doing it inadvertently, but I don't actually think that's what people intend to do at all. But our education teaches us to not see, to repress discomfort, to suppress, to follow the party line… For me, the personal is political, it's physiological, it's psychological and needs to involve the planet. So that means finding a way to tell our stories and story-telling itself (or poetry) as part of that. I would say that's quite a distinct or radical departure from traditional dietetics.

How did you get into this work? How did you come to this understanding?

J: How did you come to this work?

L: I think that my political awakening came… I can say two main things. [My experience] in the mental health system…and just seeing how there was no vocabulary and certainly no theoretical framework for it. And at the same time, when I couldn't work, I signed up to a literature and women's studies course. At about the same time, I got a critical framework of sorts. That was hugely instrumental in change.

What do you think dietitians' roles in social justice should or could be? What do we need to do differently?

J: What should or could dietitians' roles be in social justice?

L: Our practice has to be grounded in our commitment to social justice. If it doesn't, it's grounded in a commitment to oppression. And that's not ethical. So, we need to get real about this. If we want a healthy society, we need a fair society. In a fair society, we have to be actively challenging injustice. We need to get ourselves trained up on it. We need to have conversations.

J: What do we need? You mentioned how you were trained as a dietitian. What, then, do we need to do differently?

L: When I'm training dietitians, we think "I have to do this because it's policy" or "we have to do this". It implies that they're caught; their hands are tied. They're not even questioning it. Why would they? As a first step, we have to create a space where we name these things. We have to name oppression; we have to keep on naming it. We always have a choice and there are always consequences.

We do need a vocabulary for change… The non-communicable diseases— these are power-related diseases—, we need to start calling them that! We need to be aware of power dynamics and to decolonize education. And that starts with naming and disrupting power hierarchies and making knowledge situated and embodied.

J: How does this inform the work that you do now?

L: Relatively recently, I realized that… I had to be radical in my work. That I need to look into the deep root of the problem to find the deep root of change. Since I've realized that, what's changed in my work is putting more energy into spoken word performances and seeing what huge impact that has and speaking more explicitly…asking questions like "when is it okay to advocate and approach things as neoliberal". The answer is, never! So, to stop trying to tweak things and salvage things that remain neoliberal… The strategy is build what you do want. Keep moving! What I've learned more recently is to disrupt and build. Analysis, vision, strategy. That's not mine, that's someone else's template. But when I heard it more recently, I thought "yeah, that's it". If we think of it as just dietetics, we're doing ourselves a disservice! We're teaching a revolution. Our vehicle is dietetics, but it's bigger than that. It has bigger implications; it's a political project. Education is a political project. We can either teach prejudice-based medicine or we dismantle the status quo. You can't have it both ways!

Gloria Lucas

Tell me about your work.

G: I started Nalgona Positivity Pride (NPP) about 5 years ago. NPP is a Xicana-brown body-positive organization that focuses on eating disorders, awareness in communities of colour, intersectional body positivity, and the link between colonialism and eating disorders. We currently run three different support groups and programme for people of colour who are affected by disordered eating or poor body image. I am also a public speaker and travel internationally to provide education to different communities. NPP is also my small business where we provide an array of different merchandise that serve to continue our purpose.

When I was going trying to gain sense of my own disorder, I wanted to know why I had developed an eating disorder. I was unable to find that answer. Everything that I was reading did not really speak for me, and that's how I delved into historical trauma and epigenetics and how colonialism has fractured our self-esteem, body image, and our relationship with food.

NPP was an urgent effort to create unique advocacy and resources for Indigenous people and people of colour who struggle with eating disorders (ED). Considering the large gap that exists in the professional eating disorders' world for meeting the needs of Indigenous people and people of colour, I knew it was important for me to create something where my own healing could be supported. I am a strong believer of our community members creating our own opportunities for healing—away from institutions that are racist and have historically harmed us. NPP has served as my own medicine for my healing. My goal for next year is to collect the stories of brown women and Indigenous descent women who have struggled with eating disorders. You never hear those stories, and invisibility is violence. The fact that I was not able to distinguish my own eating disorder because I wasn't able to see someone like myself is violence. It's time that we uncover our stories and we support one another.

J: How have you found colonialism and trauma to be impacting people's relationships with food and their bodies?

G: There are many ways that colonialism impacts people of colour. We need to acknowledge that colonialism never ended and it continues to impact marginalized communities. For instance, communities of colour and Indigenous communities continue to be disproportionately affected by food deserts and environmental racism. Environmental racism exists because white supremacy has informed all of us that our lives and our quality of life don't matter because we are not human. White supremacy and all the beliefs that came with white supremacy were violently introduced the moment Europeans touched native land and conquered Indigenous peoples and land.

So, when you think about 500 years of ongoing racism, sexual violence, environmental degradation, transphobia, poverty, displacement, and cultural genocide, there is no way the survivors of this lineage cannot be affected. It is impossible to completely erase those traumas. More and more the study of epigenetics is informing us of how trauma in previous generations impact DNA and cellular matter for the following generations. Not to mention, mental health, coping skills, and learned behaviours have been shaped by colonialism and historical trauma across generations.

The moment Europeans stepped foot on this continent, it impacted local ecosystems, spiritualities, language, and more. Yet there's no acknowledgement of our history because schools are not teaching the correct history; our families don't know the stories because of cultural genocide and white supremacy and on top of how we've lost the ability to talk about feelings and emotions because of the hardships of colonialism. The little acknowledgement that does exist is not enough to make people understand the complexities of historical trauma in our families.

Through colonialism, the culture of food changed. Europeans introduced sheep, cows, pigs, and more. Colonialism changed Indigenous peoples' diets from plant based to animal based. Slavery as well as colonialism made Indigenous peoples dependent on Spanish food. All through Latin America,

"Europeanization" was rewarded, and that also changed Indigenous people's relationship with native foods. Rape, acculturation, structural violence, and slavery resulted in the blend of these cuisines and have led to Central American food, soul food, Mexican food, etc.

Colonialism also changed medicine and ceremony. According to the essay, "The Modern/Colonial Food System in a Paradigm of War", amaranth was a ceremonial plant for the Mexican people. When Europeans came, they stigmatized that plant and destroyed all amaranth plants they could find. If anyone was found with just one seed of amaranth, their hands would be chopped off. We see this serving as a tactic of cultural genocide.

According to Dr. Linda Alvarez from the Food Empowerment Project, for Europeans, food was a cultural, religious, and class identifier. In other words, food was a performative matter. Europeans saw native foods as subordinate foods; they believed that if they ate native foods, then they would become inferior like native peoples. This is where the belief of "good" foods and "bad" foods comes from. Conclusively, diet culture is a product of colonialism. Native people were highly spiritual and their ceremonies were based a lot on ritual and land. Colonialism robbed Indigenous people from spirituality and ceremony. When the disruption happened with land, so came a disruption with self-esteem and our identity. Women, alongside two-spirit individuals, lost identity, power, direct access to the supernatural world, and community positions. When you lose your humanity and your relationship with the land, it's bound to hurt your relationship with food. It also accounted for the enslavement of men to work in mines in South America. The essay, *A Flood of Tears and Blood: And Yet the Pope said Indians Had Souls* by Eduardo Galeano, states that Bolivian Indian miners, "for the few coins they would receive for their work, the Indians bought coca leafs instead of food: chewing it, they could -at the price of shortening their lives- better endure the deadly takes imposed on them. In addition to coca the Indians drank potent aguardiente and burn their guts with pure alcohol as sterile forms of revenge for the condemned".

If we know that (1) Indigenous peoples engaged in disordered eating and that that there is a genetic link with eating disorders and (2) there is a connection between food insecurity and eating disorder, then we can understand why people of colour and Indigenous people develop eating disorders. Furthermore, historical trauma, racist beauty ideals, displacement, and the continual oppression of women and queer folks do not help.

What does social justice mean to you?

J: What does social justice mean to you?

G: Social justice means that marginalized people's experiences are centred. The universal narrative from the last 500 years has been of white, privileged, able-bodied, heterosexual, cis-gendered people. It's time to shift that, and it's time to start centering the experiences of marginalized people. For white people to take a step back and for people of colour and Indigenous peoples to empower each other. Social justice does not mean for white people to save us. We are capable of saving ourselves. I don't want white folks speaking for me.

We all have privilege, and the way we can be allies to those that don't share the same accessibility is to listen to them and when wanted to offer a platform, space, or resource for that story to be heard. Additionally, in order for social justice to exist, we need to change academia and the way we perceive credibility. Why do people with letters after their last name get to speak on matters that don't pertain to them? As far as I'm concerned, only people who have lived that life can speak about that life. Because it is our story, it is our narrative. White people have been trying to tell our stories on their own terms forever, and it just perpetuates injury... Also, for the people with privilege, always ask yourself, "Am I doing more than harm than good by participating in this? Am I taking away another person's place?" I recently saw a film about fatphobia where a lot of thin people took up space in the film. There are enough fat people in the world that can speak for themselves.

How did you get into this work? How did you come to this understanding?

J: How did you come to form Nalgona and start doing this work?

G: I didn't expect NPP to blow up and be what it is today. To be honest I was not sure what I was creating. There were no models for me to follow to get a clear understanding of what I wanted NPP to be down the line. I see it as something I was meant to do for my ancestors. Ultimately this is what many folks who are building movements and shifts from a marginalized background have to do; we create our own opportunities. We are very resilient and creative people that can create a lot with very little.

What do you think dietitians' roles in social justice should or could be? What do we need to do differently?

J: What has the reception been among dietitians on your work?

G: I think that dietitians have, for the most part, been wanting this information. They know that there's a need for it, and there is a lack of training and knowledge. Like all people who are in a position of helping many, check what your biases are; change them. Also, become aware of the possibility that you yourself might also be struggling with disordered eating. Eating disorders in this field is very high.

J: I had mentioned to you that part of the purpose of this interview is to showcase the work that you're doing. I'm interested in hearing what being an ally as a dietitian would mean. What would you want to tell dietitians about being an ally?

G: Studying how colonialism impacted food to better understand their patients. Understanding the concept of decolonizing their diet... Also, acknowledging the privilege that one has. We all have privilege! I'm able-bodied. I'm heterosexual. I'm able to quit my job and do this full time. I was born in this country. Acknowledging all these privileges that we have so that we can face the reality that we might not understand our clients 100%. That is helpful. Doing a lot of listening is important and trying to support those already doing the work... If you see research, ask yourself, "where was this research done? Which population? Where?"... One of my friends had a dietitian tell them that Mexican food was unhealthy. Please unlearn and dismantle all racism. Also, study historical trauma and post-traumatic slave syndrome. Food is political and it's so tied to identity and dietitians need to honour that... Are your services friendly to working-class people? How many fat clients do you have and why? We also need to recognize that health varies from person to person. Become more sensitive to folks who are low-income, homeless, have chronic illness, and who face other obstacles that makes it very difficult to be your definition of "healthy".

Conclusion

A final question that I wish to address is one that troubles the very premise of this chapter: Does advocacy lay beyond the scope of dietitians' knowledge and practice? For some, the answer is "yes". In this view, advocacy is too far afield of the professions' core commitment to the application of nutrition science in promoting and treating health.[4] For me, however, the answer is "no". While the science of food and nutrition is a foundation of dietetic knowledge and practice, it does not comprise the entirety of our knowledge and practice, nor is it mutually exclusive with the pursuit of social justice through advocacy. Rather, science is but one pillar of our knowledge and practice that is essential to what dietitians have to offer to the struggle for health equity and social justice. Nutrition science, when complemented by other ways of knowing, is an important component in understanding, challenging, and changing social problems. As Trevor Hancock (2015) writes, *Advocacy: It's not a dirty word, it's a duty* (p. E86).

Moving forward, I am confident that as a profession, we have the capacity to find creative ways to draw on our proficiency in nutrition science and work collaboratively with others whose knowledge and experience span other areas of expertise and experience. What is more, I assert that, as a profession—a group of individuals who have benefit of the gifts of higher education, professional employment, and other social and economic privilege—we have a responsibility to use our knowledge and expertise to make the world a more equitable, just place. In other words, we have a responsibility as a profession, and as individual practitioners, because we have "response ability"—the ability to respond, to health inequities and social injustices. In the end, the problems that we face, from social and economic inequities to the pending devastation of climate change, and the devastating impacts that these

---

[4] The ICDA defines a dietitian-nutritionist as "A professional who applies the science of food and nutrition to promote health, prevent and treat disease to optimise the health of individuals, groups, communities and populations" (ICDA 2017).

have on health, are too great and too demanding of everyone's capacity to create change, to absolve ourselves from doing so.

Assignments

1. Based on this chapter and on your own experience, how would you define social justice and health equity from a nutrition perspective? What principles, knowledge, skills, and actions might be necessary to support dietitians' roles in social justice advocacy?
2. Think about a social justice or equity issue that is relevant to the community in which you live. Reflect on how and why this issue might be of concern for dietitians. How might this issue impact community members' ability to access safe, affordable food in a dignified and sustainable way? How might this issue impact people's nutritional, cultural, emotional, social, psychological, and spiritual health? What might you do as a future or current dietitian to get involved in your community to address this issue?
3. Advocacy doesn't have to take a lot of time or resources to effect change. One small action that you can take to effect change is writing a letter to a local, provincial, regional, or national elected official on an issue you care about. Remember to identify and properly address the most appropriate individual for the issue, be cordial, and be sure to ask for the specific change you want to see happen to address this issue.

Definition of Keywords and Terms

Activism	Direct action, such as protests, demonstrations, or acts of civil disobedience, aimed at bringing about social or political change.
Advocacy	Actions by individuals, groups, or organizations that aim to influence or create change regarding an issue by raising awareness, building networks, and fostering support by others.
Classism	Classism is a form of systemic oppression based on a persons' or groups' perceived socio-economic class which comprises a complex mix of material wealth and social status, as well as education, customs, attitudes, behaviours, values, and appearance. Class-based oppression is also associated with class privilege for those of higher material wealth and social status. Classism intersects with other forms of oppression, such as racism and sex-

	ism, to inform an individuals' or groups' social standing along multiple axes (i.e. race, gender, class).
Colonialism	Colonialism is an ongoing process whereby one group of people subjugates and exploits another group of people through overt and covert policies and practices including war, annexing land, and constructing the subjugated group as inferior and deserving or in need of the colonizing groups' control.
Health equity	Like social justice, health equity is multifaceted but in essence describes the conceptualization of social justice vis a vis health.
Power-related diseases/illness	Aphramor (2016) describes power-related illnesses as health and nutrition problems that are largely the result of social injustice rather than inherent deficits among clients and their communities but that are often understood and acted upon, such as through health promotion and nutrition education efforts, to be the result of individuals' poor choices.
Racism	Racism is a form of systemic oppression based on the belief that race is a biological characteristic and that some races are innately inferior. Racism is also associated with race-based privilege, namely, white privilege, whereby white people are afforded unearned or undue status in society. Racism intersects with other forms of oppression, such as classism and sexism, to inform an individuals' or groups' social standing along multiple axes (i.e. race, gender, class).
Sexism	Sexism is a form of system oppression that devalues individuals, groups, knowledge, practices, and ways of being that are associated with femininity. Sexism is also associated with gender-based privilege, namely, male privilege. Sexism intersects with other forms of oppression, such as classism and racism, to inform an individuals' or groups' social standing along multiple axes (i.e. race, gender, class).
Social justice	Although defined in various ways, at its core, social justice describes a state of social, structural, environmental, and political fairness that promotes equitable distribution of material and representational power and that redresses historical injustices.

Structural competence   Structural competence describes knowledge and
                                      skill-based knowledge on how to redress structural
                                      inequities such as those caused by gender-, race-,
                                      and class-based oppression.

How This Chapter Addresses the Critical Dietetic Framework

This chapter addresses all of the elements of the critical dietetic framework. The
first and third elements of the critical dietetic framework are addressed in this chapter which draws on multi- and transdisciplinary literature, as well as interviews with
individuals whose work is informed by variously situated perspectives including
academic, performance poet, dietitian, community activist, eating disorder survivor,
and person of colour, to understand elaborate meanings of social justice and health
equity. One of the core concepts of this chapter is that social justice and health
equity require reflexive engagement to work through the complex and sometimes
contradictory, political commitments of these concepts. The fourth element of the
critical dietetic framework is addressed by another key concern of this chapter. That
is, dietitians could and should play a central role as advocates and activists in
advancing social justice through social and political change.

References

Aphramor L (2016) Glossary. Available via http://lucyaphramor.com/dietitian/glossary/. Accessed
    15 July 2018
Aphramor L, Asada Y, Atkins J, et al (2009) Critical dietetics: a declaration. Practice 48:1–2.
    Available via https://criticaldieteticsblog.files.wordpress.com/2011/10/critical-dietetics-decla-
    ration.pdf. Accessed 23 Apr 2018
Birkenmaier J (2003) On becoming a social justice practitioner. Soc Thought 22(2–3):41–54
Brady J (2017) Trading the apron for the white lab coat: a contemporary history of dietetics in
    Canada, 1954 to 2016. Dissertation, Queen's University
Braveman P (2006) Health disparities and health equity: concepts and measurement. Annu Rev
    Public Health 27:167–194
Buettner-Schmidt K, Lobo ML (2012) Social justice: a concept analysis. J Adv Nurs 68(4):948–958
Canadian Nurses Association (2010) Social justice: a means to an end, an end in itself. Available
    via   https://www.cna-aiic.ca/~/media/cna/page-content/pdf-en/social_justice_2010_e.pdf.
    Accessed 18 November 2018
Duckworth V, Maxwell B (2015) Extending the mentor role in initial teacher education: embracing
    social justice. Int J Mentor Coach Educ 4(1):4–20
Duff WM, Flinn A, Suurtamm KE, Wallace DA (2013) Social justice impact of archives: a prelimi-
    nary investigation. Arch Sci 13:317–348
DuPuis M, Harrison JL, Goodman D (2011) Just food? In: Alkon AH, Agyeman J (eds) Cultivating
    food justice: race, class, and sustainability. MIT Press, Cambridge, MA, pp 283–308
Dharamsi S, MacEntee MI (2002) Dentistry and distributive justice. Soc Sci Med, 55:323–329
Hancock T (2015) Advocacy: it's not a dirty word, it's a duty. Can J Public Health 106(3):E86–E88

Hansen H, Braslow J, Rohrbaugh RM (2017) From cultural to structural competency training psychiatry residents to act on social determinants of health and institutional racism. JAMA Psychiatry 75(2):117–118

International Confederation of Dietetic Associations (2017) Definition of dietitian-nutritionist. https://www.internationaldietetics.org/Downloads/International-Definition-of-Dietitian.aspx. Accessed 16 Feb 2018

Kirmayer LJ, Kronick R, Rousseau C (2018) Advocacy as key to structural competency in psychiatry. JAMA Psychiatry 75(2):119–120

Metzl JM, Hansen H (2014) Structural competency: theorizing a new medical engagement with stigma and inequality. Soc Sci Med 103:126–133

Mikkonen J, Raphael D (2010) Social determinants of health: the Canadian facts. Available via http://thecanadianfacts.org. Accessed 24 Apr 2018

Peter F (2001) Health equity and social justice. J Appl Philos 18(2):159–170

Public Health Agency of Canada (2017) Glossary of terms. Available via http://www.phac-aspc. gc.ca/php-psp/ccph-cesp/glos-eng.php#e. Accessed 31 Jan 2018

Raine K (2014) Improving nutritional health of the public through social change: finding our roles in collective action. Can J Diet Pract Res 75(3):160–164

Rodriguez JC (2010) Advocacy is a natural part of our life and work. J Am Diet Assoc 110(11):1604

Sandretto S, Ballard K, Burke P, Kane R, Lang C, Schon P, Whyte B (2007) Nailing jello to the wall: articulating conceptualizations of social justice. Teach Teach Theory Pract 13(3):307–322

Scott B, Wainwright Counts E, Medora M, Woolery C (1998) The dietitian's role in ending world hunger: as citizen and health professional. Top Clin Nutr 13(4): 31–45

Van Soest D (1992) Peace and social justice as an integral part of the social work curriculum: a North American perspective. Australian Social Work 45(1):29–38

World Health Organization (2010) A conceptual framework for action on the social determinants of health: social determinates of health discussion paper 2. Available via http://www.who.int/social_determinants/corner/SDHDP2.pdf. Accessed 22 Mar 2018

Whitehead M (1992) The concepts and principles of equity in health. Int J Health Ser 22(3):429–445

Further Reading

Biltekoff C (2013) Eating right in America: the cultural politics of food and health. Duke University Press, Durham, NC

Birkenmaier J (2003) On becoming a social justice practitioner. Soc Thought 22(2–3):41–54

Hayes-Conroy A, Hayes-Conroy J (2013) Doing nutrition differently: critical approaches to diet and dietary intervention. Routledge, New York

Laverack G (2013) Health activism: foundations and strategies. Sage, Los Angeles

Raine K (2014) Improving nutritional health of the public through social change: finding our roles in collective action. Can J Diet Pract Res 75(3):160–164

Glossary

Activism Direct action, such as protests, demonstrations or acts of civil disobedience, aimed at bringing about social or political change.

Advocacy Actions by individuals, groups or organizations that aim to influence or create change regarding an issue by raising awareness, building networks and fostering support by others.

Agribusiness Is the business of agricultural production. The term was coined in 1957 by Goldberg and Davis. It includes agrichemicals, breeding, crop production (farming and contract farming), distribution, farm machinery, processing and seed supply, as well as marketing and retail sales. All agents of the food and fibre value chain and those institutions that influence it are part of the agribusiness system.

Ampowerment Refers to a meaningful sense of one's power from within (Aphramor 2016). The term ampowerment is coined by Lucy Aphramor. As Aphramor explains, "Lifestyle change falls under the rubric of ampowerment, which relates to self-care. Ampowerment fosters empowerment through links with a critical awareness of power-over, and increased capacity to engage in and influence power-with relationships. Empowerment is a process that involves systemic social change, with action preceded by collective consciousness raising. It does not stop at self-esteem. It is not about compliance or co-ercion" (Aphramor 2016).

Anti-oppression Anti-oppression is an approach or paradigm that is rooted in ending systemic oppression of all kinds, including but not limited to, racism, sexism, classism, homo- and transphobia, sizeism and so on.

Axiology Axiology is the study of what is valued or what is considered to be of value. Critical dietetic axiology comprises the approaches, knowledges, political commitments and practices that form the central core of critical dietetics.

Big food Refers to the transnational food and beverage industry that is powerful, profit driven and focused on the manufacture of ultra-processed foods with serious consequences for public health and the environment.

© Springer Nature Switzerland AG 2019
J. Coveney, S. Booth (eds.), *Critical Dietetics and Critical Nutrition Studies*,
Food Policy, https://doi.org/10.1007/978-3-030-03113-8

Capitalism A system of economics based on the private ownership of capital and production inputs and on the production of goods and services for profit.

Civic agriculture "The emergence and growth of community-based agriculture and food production activities that not only meet consumer demands for fresh, safe, and locally produced foods but create jobs, encourage entrepreneurship, and strengthen community identity" (Lyson, 1999, p.2).

Civic dietetics Civic dietetics is the application of dietetics to enhance public health by addressing food system structures, impacts and policies and their relationship to food choices (Wilkins, Lapp, et.al. 2010).

Class society *The Communist Manifesto* describes the process by which society developed over time so that today it is divided into roughly two great classes. Marxists often refer to the ruling class as the bourgeoisie and the working class as the proletariat. Each class is defined by its relationship to the major means of production.

Classism Classism is a form of systemic oppression based on a persons' or groups' perceived socio-economic class which comprises a complex mix of material wealth and social status, as well as education, customs, attitudes, behaviours, values and appearance. Class-based oppression is also associated with class privilege for those of higher material wealth and social status. Classism intersects with other forms of oppression, such as racism and sexism, to inform an individuals' or groups' social standing along multiple axes (i.e. race, gender, class).

Colonialism Colonialism is an ongoing process, whereby one group of people subjugates and exploits another group of people through overt and covert policies and practices including war, annexing land and constructing the subjugated group as inferior and deserving or in need of the colonizing groups' control.

Critical praxis Praxis was first defined by scholar-activist Paulo Freire (2012) as "reflection and action directed at the structures to be transformed" (p. 32). For critical dietetics, critical praxis comprises the expression of the insights garnered by critical social theory through action for social justice.

Critical To be critical is to question the way things are so as to enhance or expand upon established epistemologies (ways of knowing) and bodies of knowledge. Often being critical is taken to be negative, but this is not a complete understanding. To be critical is to seek to transform and grow ways of thinking about any particular topic.

Discourse "A series of representations, practices, and performances through which meanings are produced, connected into networks, and legitimized. Discourses are heterogeneous, regulated, embedded, situated, and performative" (Gingras 2009, p. 238).

Disenchantment The move away from more mystical forms of belief towards a rational, secular approach to organizing social groups. In this context, the term owes an intellectual debt to nineteenth-century sociologist, Max Weber, who employed the term to explain the move in western cultures towards bureaucratic and modernized forms of rationalism.

Ecological nutrition A term used to capture such a multidimensional and systems approach now broadly considered necessary to achieving *sustainable diets*.

Epistemology Epistemology is a concept that describes the various ways of understanding what counts as knowledge. There are many epistemologies. Mainstream dietetic knowledge and practice is informed by positivist epistemology which understands knowledge creation as the process of uncovering truths about the world through the scientific method. Critical dietetics is informed by a post-structural epistemology wherein truth is understood as being in constant flux and knowledge creation as requiring multiple, differently situated perspectives, approaches and methods.

Ethics Principles that govern behaviours that have a strong moral foundation.

Food crime Activities encompassing economic deception and physical harms, issues of personal health and fraudulent activities such as food substitution, adulteration and misrepresentation (Croall, 2007).

Food democracy Food democracy is the counterweight to the industrial food system. It can be considered a movement that seeks to create alternative food systems to improve health and transform passive consumers into active food citizens.

Forms of power Forms of power refer to the many ways that power is a factor in social relationships. These include one's position within an organization, historical contribution(s) (of oneself or one's family members), expertise or authority, serving as a funding decision-maker (deciding who or what projects get funded and by how much), determining who has decision-making authority (including who has a voice, to what voices to attend and how messages will be conveyed), one's personal or one's group's physical force or strength, gender, wealth, recognition and notoriety and positional power (e.g. the teacher-student relationship) (Wartenberg, 1991).

Gastronomy The appreciation of the art and knowledge of food and cooking. In this chapter, gastronomic has been used to refer to the use of senses and experience in food choice.

Globalization Bosses and bourgeois politicians talk about globalization as if it is a new and benign form of capitalism that peacefully spreads wealth and stability to poor countries around the world. But the truth is that what the mainstream media calls globalization is just a modern form of imperialism. Now, instead of colonizing oppressed countries through the brute force of imperialist armies alone, bankers and corporations use institutions like the World Bank and the International Monetary Fund to help coerce those countries into bending to their will.

Health equity Like social justice, health equity is multifaceted but in essence describes the conceptualization of social justice vis-a-vis health.

Ideology Refers, traditionally, to the relatively stable and enduring sense that a person has of ones' identity, such as gender, sexual orientation, ethnicity and class (Lee, Sammon & Dumbrill 2007).

Imperialism Imperialism is the final stage of capitalism that is reached when the capitalists of a particular country are compelled to economically expand beyond their own borders through military force or other methods of coercion.

Individualism Refers to the conception of an individual being the essential proprietor of one's own capacities, owing nothing to society for them (Macpherson 1962).

Intersectionality Intersectionality was coined by feminist legal scholar Kimberle Crenshaw (1991) to describe the ways in which the experience of and social structures supporting one form of oppression vary when intersecting with other forms of oppression.

Microaggression Microaggressions comprise the subtle everyday intended or unintended acts, such as direct verbal harassment or misrepresentation in the media, which collectively contribute to the social exclusion of oppressed groups.

NAFTA The North American Free Trade Agreement is an agreement signed by Canada, Mexico and the United States, creating a trilateral trade bloc in North America.

Narrative A story or account of events, interactions and experiences that are selectively recalled, arranged and interpreted by a person, family or community. Narratives serve to organize and give meaning to the storyteller(s) (Lee, Sammon & Dumbrill 2007).

Nutritionism Scrinis (2013) coined the term to describe the shifting focus towards the specific nutrients in food as providing some health benefits and the resulting emphasis by consumers to purchase food on this basis instead of other aspects such as taste, cost or sociocultural meaning.

Ontology A philosophical term referring to the way things exist or are being. In this chapter the term is used to highlight the ways in which food and nourishment support growth and development of physical things (bodies) but also abstract things like mental and spiritual existence.

Ontology Refers to the branch of philosophy that deals with being (Lee, Sammon & Dumbrill 2007).

Other Refers to the attempt to form a personal or group identity, where comparison of ourselves to others creates an understanding of ourselves as separate and different from others. The process of comparison can establish identity but can also create a sense of superiority and an objectification of those who are "different" (Lee, Sammon & Dumbrill 2007).

Post-oppositional perspective Ways of working and engaging that move beyond being in opposition, that is, working collaboratively rather than counter to whomever or whatever one considers as the antagonist. Working from a post-oppositional perspective, one embraces interconnectivity and creates conditions for fruitful dialogues towards transformational possibilities. One considers political, ethical, social, spiritual, intellectual and pedagogical dimensions of issues. Keating (2013) declared that post-oppositionality "calls for and enacts innovative, radically inclusionary ways of reading, teaching, and communicating".

Power-related diseases/illness Aphramor (2016) describes power-related illnesses as health and nutrition problems that are largely the result of social injustice rather than inherent deficits among clients and their communities but that are often understood and acted upon, such as through health promotion and nutrition education efforts, to be the result of individuals' poor choices.

Praxis Refers to the unity of theory and practice (Lee, Sammon & Dumbrill 2007).

Professional identity This is a concept which describes how we perceive ourselves as professionals and how we communicate that to others.

Professional socialization Socialization is the process by which individuals acquire the identity of a professional. This process involves the learning of the values, norms, behaviours and social skills associated with their profession.

Racism Racism is a form of systemic oppression based on the belief that race is a biological characteristic and that some races are innately inferior. Racism is also associated with race-based privilege, namely, white privilege, whereby white people are afforded unearned or undue status in society. Racism intersects with other forms of oppression, such as classism and sexism, to inform an individuals' or groups' social standing along multiple axes (i.e. race, gender, class).

Reflexivity Understood to be different from reflection in that reflection can involve an actor examining an object, whereas reflexivity is an internal conversation where an embodied actor in a social context bends their thoughts back on themselves (Vink, et al., 2017).

Reflexivity When one is practising reflexivity, she is going beyond reflecting on an experience and how she can improve practice as a result. Reflexivity involves exploring one's feelings, motives and reactions to a situation and how this influences her thinking about that situation.

Scientism A belief that science and the scientific method is the only way of understanding natural or social phenomena. This chapter has used the term scientistic to refer to a preference for scientific method and proof.

Sexism Sexism is a form of system oppression that devalues individuals, groups, knowledge, practices and ways of being that are associated with femininity. Sexism is also associated with gender-based privilege, namely, male privilege. Sexism intersects with other forms of oppression, such as classism and racism, to inform an individuals' or groups' social standing along multiple axes (i.e. race, gender, class).

Social justice Although defined in various ways, at its core, social justice describes a state of social, structural, environmental and political fairness that promotes equitable distribution of material and representational power and that redresses historical injustices.

Standardized dietitian The process by which professional education and professional practices inculcate a particular standardized subjectivity.

Structural competence Structural competence describes knowledge- and skill-based know-how to redress structural inequities such as those caused by gender-, race- and class-based oppression.

Sustainable diets The FAO and Bioversity International define sustainable diets as "… those diets with low environmental impacts which contribute to food and nutrition security and to healthy life for present and future generations. Sustainable diets are protective and respectful of biodiversity and ecosystems, culturally acceptable, accessible, economically fair and affordable; nutritionally adequate, safe and healthy; while optimizing natural and human resources" (Burlingame and Dernini 2012).

Sustainable food systems The Food and Agriculture Organization (FAO) defines SFS as those that "…[deliver] food and nutrition security for all in such a way that the economic, social and environmental bases to generate food security and nutrition for future generations are not compromised" (HLPE 2017).

To be powered over To be subject to the forms of power that another person or organization holds and wields.

To have power over To exercise one's power over another or a group in a social relationship.

Transdisciplinary Is the bringing together of different disciplines to offer a more complex and nuanced understanding of a topic, whereby the disciplines themselves are enhanced in the process. Transdisciplinary is different from multi- or interdisciplinary scholarship, in that the latter describes a process of bringing various disciplinary perspectives to bear on a topic, in this case, dietetic education, research and practice, whereby dietetics is transformed and enhanced.

Transformative practice This is a way of practising that results in beneficial change.

Index

Printed in the United States
By Bookmasters